THE DARK SIDE OF STATINS

by

Duane Graveline, M.D., M.P.H.

New and Expanded Edition: August 2017

Published by Spacedoc Media, LLC.

www.spacedoc.com

The information and opinions in this book are based upon the author's personal and professional experiences and research. Information in this book is not intended to be a substitute for professional medical advice and care. Always consult with a qualified medical professional before making medication, supplement, or lifestyle changes or decisions.

Dietary supplements reviewed in this book have not been evaluated by the United States Food and Drug Administration for the possible benefits described.

Information in this book is not intended to diagnose, treat, cure or prevent any disease.

Active ingredients in dietary supplements can vary greatly between brands and manufacturers.

3

CONTENTS

4

,

Foreword
by Glyn Wainwright

This book is an exposé of the current, powerfully marketed myth that we can fix, or even prevent, certain of our health problems by consuming a reductase inhibitor — better known to all as a statin.

Statins are 'toxic medicines' that claim to save us by attacking our ability to synthesize those very things that sustain and repair us in our daily lives, the products of our naturally evolved metabolism. Dr. Graveline describes a celebrated metabolic system known to biochemists as our 'Mevalonate Metabolic Pathway', and the problems that arise from attempting to blockade this vital process from taking place in every living cell in our bodies.

Everyone who has experience with statins or cares for someone who has been damaged by statins needs to understand the issues and testimony documented within. Dr. Graveline uses a powerful mix of descriptive explanations, case reports and scientific research references to inform everyone from lay-person to expert.

He exposes a grave historic error in our interpretation of the role of fats and lipids in heart disease. This failed statin 'miracle cure' was based upon the false premise that fats and cholesterol, a major factor in the evolution of complex cells and animals, suddenly became a bad thing in the late 20th Century.

Having something for everyone, this book will inform those who have experienced adverse reactions to statin drugs and those involved as family, friends and caregivers.

There is discussion and guidance of dietary changes and supplements, which may help to mitigate the more extreme damage done by statins. Understanding the damage to mitochondria, coenzyme Q10, cholesterol, dolichols and the protective role of antioxidants is an important step in addressing the damage.

Guidance to medical doctors regarding statin adverse effects encourages the sympathetic discussion of these adverse reactions. The case reports in this book show the many ways in which statins can impact the lives of patients. The extensive personal testimony collected by Dr. Graveline is a measured and emotionally powerful perspective on the public's response to the stain crisis.

These patients' accounts of adverse effects should be taken very seriously by health professionals. They should be used to confront the powerful corporations who have misguidedly promoted ever-wider use of statins, and to expose the often devastating consequences of long-term mevalonate blockade

In this fourth book in the series, Dr. Graveline pays particular attention to the damage done by statins to our mitochondrial DNA, the parts of each cell which converts metabolic energy into cellular power known as adenosine triphosphate (ATP). Our mitochondrial DNA is normally protected by the products of the mevalonate metabolic pathway.

It is poignant and disturbing that, having discovered the devastation of cholesterol lowering drugs, many patients continue to seek other ways of reducing their cholesterol levels.

It is important to combat the corporate promotion of the erroneous and harmful myth of 'bad' cholesterol. The consequence of this error is extensive statin generated damage to all tissues and mitochondrial function in particular, as explored here by Dr. Graveline.

Glyn Wainwright
MSc MBCS CEng CITP

Preface

Tens of thousands of statin users have complained to their doctors of weakness, instability, easy fatigue, muscle aches and pains, burning of their extremities, depression and faulty memory, to which their doctors generally have responded, "You have to expect this now. You are over fifty."

Although these experienced doctors have all pointed to a correct presumptive diagnosis, few have been entirely comfortable with this explanation because of a curious recurring element in their presentation. All have been on statins of one brand or another and the transition from midlife vigor to the multiple infirmities of the elderly has been much too swift in most of these cases.

In the few months since the previous office visit, an aura of senescence has evolved in these patients. Doctors deal with the presence of aging on a daily basis and are acutely sensitive to its telltale first traces. All of us are vulnerable to aging but the timing here just doesn't feel right.

Somehow the word 'timing' seems to be the key and our minds finally jump to the correct interpretation. The complaints their patients are reporting may be common, even routine, in the elderly yet these people are for the most part in their fifties, sixties and seventies, and sometimes even much younger.

If anything out of the ordinary can be attributed to these complaints of faulty memory, weakness and various aches and pains, it is because of their prematurity — premature aging.

Conditions are being complained about that ordinarily would not be seen until much later in life. Are these statin users being robbed of their "golden years"? Is it possible that their passage to old age has been expedited? If so, what could be the mechanism?

In recent years, I have learned that the oxidizing tendency of the air we breathe, with its production of highly energetic radicals from our foodstuffs, has necessitated the evolution in our bodies of powerful antioxidant systems to minimize the oxidative damage to our tissues and, more importantly, our mitochondrial DNA.

This book will take you on a journey where many doctors really do not want to go — not after decades of prescribing statins. The truth is something few of us wish to hear, not if it means we have been wrong for almost 30 years of use, during which time the drug companies have been subtly updating their statin drug adverse effects warnings.

Would any of you care to look at a statin warning today and compare it with what they said about the same drug when first marketed? Much of what I write about in this book is now in drug company warnings.

The very idea that my practice philosophy was wrong for many years is very difficult for me to accept; and to think I was following the dictates of our national leadership, marching in lockstep with most of you to the misguided fallacy of cholesterol causation of heart disease.

We should never have been taking statins without also taking CoQ10. For many who have experienced problems with statins, much of it could have been prevented, but the situation is not hopeless.

I have included in this book my thoughts on the combined benefits of proper diet and supplements to help restore mitochondrial function and glimpse the promise of even more specific supplement use in the future.

The first chapter is by my fellow THINCS (The International Network of Cholesterol Skeptics) member

Glyn Wainwright. In this book, I first wanted to cover the critical role that cholesterol plays in human health. Glyn's excellent illustrated summary — The Wonder of Cholesterol — was perfect for this, and he kindly allowed me to use it in this book.

The rest of the book is my own material and covers the side effects of statin drugs, with special emphasis on the impact on our cell mitochondria. Some chapters cover material that is inevitably difficult to understand. There is no simple way to describe complex biochemical processes. To help, I have included a summary at the end of each chapter that covers the main points in easy to understand bullet points.

The use of statins has resulted in compromise of the vital CoQ10 and dolichol elements of our antioxidant system, resulting in seriously increased oxidative damage and mitochondrial DNA mutations.

The logical consequence of this is mitochondrial failure — insufficient mitochondria to supply the energy needs of the cell. The cell must die, and with sufficient cell death comes tissue failure.

So if it is a nerve cell, we have lost it, and perhaps thousands more, helping to explain why so much of the statin damage is permanent. The same thing holds for muscle cells. With sufficient loss of muscle cells we permanently lose muscle strength.

It is true also for the pancreas. With sufficient loss of pancreatic cells, and their insulin producing islets of Langerhans, pancreatic failure and permanent diabetes can result.

The use of statins has resulted in compromise of the dolichol and vital CoQ10 elements of our antioxidant system, resulting in seriously increased oxidative damage and DNA mutations. The logical consequence of this is premature aging. The early and progressive development of such chronic conditions of aging as muscle weakness, burning pain in the extremities, faulty coordination and failing memory — exactly the clinical picture we are seeing in tens of thousands of statin users.

Duane Graveline, M.D., M.P.H.

The Wonder of Cholesterol

by Glyn Wainwright

When you are asked to reduce your 'cholesterol level', why not ask a question which is fundamental to your health: 'Why?'

Ask "What does cholesterol do and why do we make and store so much of it in all the cells in our bodies?"
The answer is astonishingly simple: all our cells need cholesterol to function properly.

The High Cholesterol Paradox

Being told you have 'high cholesterol' is commonly taken as a sign of an unhealthy destiny. However, for many elderly people, the news that they have 'high cholesterol' is more often associated with good health and longevity.[1]
For over 50 years this has been a paradox, the 'High-Cholesterol Paradox'.
What is really going on? Let us look at the scientific facts.

Hypothesis Becomes Dogma

In the 1950s the prestigious American medical doctor, Dr Ancel Keys, supported a popular theory that heart disease was caused by dietary Fats and Cholesterol (Lipids) circulating in the blood.[2] In 1972 a British Professor, Dr John Yudkin, published a book called 'Pure, White and Deadly' which proposed over-consumption of refined sugar as the leading cause of diabetes and heart disease.[3]

The science was contested by 'interested parties', and the matter was resolved by 'government decree' in a U.S. Senate report.

On Friday January 14th 1977, Senator George McGovern's Senate Select Committee on Nutrition and Human Needs published 'Dietary Goals for the United States'.

This document sided heavily with Dr Keys' lipid theory. Thus 'hypothesis became dogma', without the benefit of scientific proof. The McGovern report recommended that we consume more carbohydrates (sugar generating foods) with more limited amounts of fats, meat and dairy. Since the 1970s there has been a rise in the use of High-Fructose Corn Syrups in processed food, and the introduction of low-fat foods which tend to have added sugar to make them attractive to eat.

Until the 1970s there had been a small but consistent percentage of overweight and obese people in the population. By the 1980s obesity rates had begun to climb significantly. This sudden acceleration of obesity is very closely associated with the adoption of new high-sugar, low-fat formulations in processed foods - the consequences of the McGovern report recommendations being adopted around the world.

Advice to reduce our intake of saturated fats, obtained from meat and dairy, caused a rise in the use of plant based oils and so-called 'vegetable fats'. This was misleadingly promoted as healthy. The biochemical destiny of dietary saturated fat is not the same as that of excess carbohydrates and sugars.

Normal Lipid Nutrition Cycle
Receptor Mediated LDL Supply to all organs

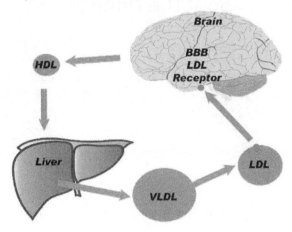

Fats do not cause obesity or disease. It is the excess sugars (glucose and fructose and refined fructose from High Fructose Corn Syrup HFCS) which create abdominal obesity.[4]

The erroneous idea, and fear, of artery-blocking fats was exploited to market fat substitutes. Invite anyone talking about 'artery-blocking fats' to hold a pat of butter in a closed fist. As the butter melts and runs out between their fingers, ask 'How do fats, which are evolved to be fluids at body temperature, block the vascular 'pipes' in our bodies?'

Plant oils are not the natural lipids for maintaining healthy human or animal cell membranes. Animal sourced fats, and essential fatty acids (EFA), are identical to those we require for the maintenance of the healthy human body.

Good Cholesterol? Bad Cholesterol?

Spot the Difference

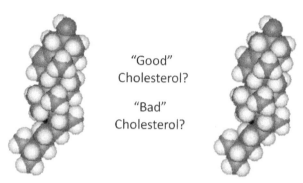

"Good"
Cholesterol?

"Bad"
Cholesterol?

A Misleading and Unscientific 'Marketing Concept'

Without exception, biochemists can confirm that all cholesterol molecules throughout the known universe are identical in every respect. So how can there be 'good' or 'bad' cholesterol. It is now possible to frighten people with unscientific descriptions like 'Good' and 'Bad' when talking about cholesterol.

This single misleading description may have prevented a whole generation from knowing the true causes of the very real disturbance in the levels of fatty nutrients (Lipids) circulating in our blood.[4]

Healthy Lipid Nutrition Cycle

The delivery of fatty nutrients is a very well-regulated cycle, a 'parcel service' of 'lipid wraps' (LDL and HDL lipid particles) circulating in the blood. These lipid wraps, HDLs and LDLs, complete with apo-protein 'labels,' assist the delivery (by receptor mediated endocytosis) of fat soluble materials and proteins from where they are sourced (the liver) to where they are needed (the organs).[7]

The measuring of these lipid wraps in your blood is used to estimate the numbers which you are given by your doctor as the 'cholesterol' level. No one really measures the cholesterol; it is merely estimated from the quantity of very useful 'lipid droplets' circulating in your blood.

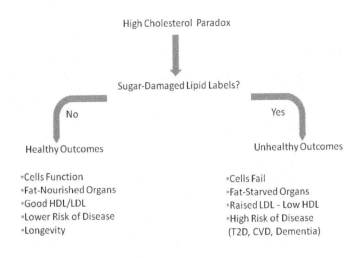

High Cholesterol Paradox

Sugar-Damaged Lipid Labels?

No — Healthy Outcomes
- Cells Function
- Fat-Nourished Organs
- Good HDL/LDL
- Lower Risk of Disease
- Longevity

Yes — Unhealthy Outcomes
- Cells Fail
- Fat-Starved Organs
- Raised LDL - Low HDL
- High Risk of Disease
 (T2D, CVD, Dementia)

These large 'lipid wraps' (LDL) have evolved to do a multitude of jobs, like transporting vital resources such as fat soluble vitamins, lipids and proteins. The cholesterol, in our lipid wraps, forms an essential part of our fatty nutrition and immune systems.

If the total blood serum cholesterol (TBSC) is high and the organs are getting enough lipids, the blood lipid circulation is healthy. The large parcels of fatty nutrients (LDL lipids) sent by the liver are consumed by our organs (receptor-mediated endocytosis) and the smaller fatty wrappers and left-over lipids (HDL Lipids) return to the liver. The Fatty Nutrients (LDL) and the recycled lipids (HDL) are in balance. Such a healthy-lipid 'high-cholesterol' person is well nourished and likely to have a long and healthy life.

Sugar-Damaged Lipid Nutrition – Broken Lipid Cycles

If the total blood serum cholesterol is high but the fatty nutrient droplets (LDLs) have sugar-damaged protein labels, the organs are unable to recognize and feed on them. The supply of fatty nutrients to organs is broken. This can happen in the decades leading up to the onset of mature-onset (type 2) diabetes.

The liver continues to supply fatty nutrients (albeit with damaged LDL labels), but the organs' receptors are unable to recognize them. The organs thus become starved of their fatty nutrients. Like badly labelled parcels in a postal service, the sugar-damaged lipids build up in the blood (raised LDL) and fewer empty wrappers are returned to the liver (low HDL).

Sugar-Damaged Lipid Cycle
LDL Labels

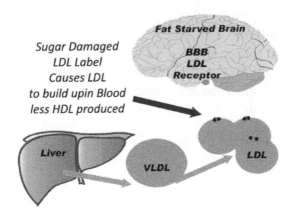

The sugar damaged LDL (erroneously called 'bad' cholesterol) in the bloodstream appears to be high. It has not been recognized by the organs that need it. It circulates in the blood, awaiting clearance by the liver. Consequently, there is less HDL (erroneously called 'good' cholesterol) to be returned by the organs.

High Cholesterol (high levels of total blood serum cholesterol TBSC) when caused by damage to the LDL lipid parcels, is a sign that lipid circulation is broken. These fats (LDL) will be scavenged to become visceral fats, deposited around the abdomen. This type of damage is associated with poor health. Our organs, such as the brain and heart, would be in a sorry state if the LDL circulating in our bloodstream was depleted or damaged.

This is where it all went wrong. In diabetics and pre-diabetics, the raised LDL was seen as overproduction and mislabeled as 'bad' cholesterol. We now know that it was a lack of consumption of LDL that caused its elevated levels in the blood, caused by Glycation (sugar attachment to lipo-proteins)

So it really doesn't matter how high your total blood serum cholesterol (TBSC) is. What really counts is the damaged condition of the blood's fatty nutrient parcels (LDL lipids). In a research review of metabolic syndromes (e.g. diabetes, heart disease, obesity, arthritis and dementia) our associates explained that the major cause of lipid damage was sugar-related.[4]

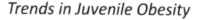

Trends in Juvenile Obesity

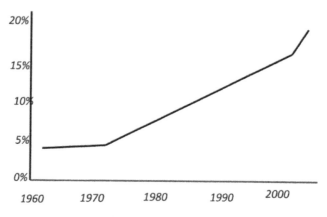

Sugar Damage (AGEs)

The abbreviation AGE (**A**dvanced **G**lycation **E**nd-product) is used to describe any sugar-damaged protein. As we age, excessive amounts of free sugars in the blood may eventually cause damage quicker than the body can repair it.[5] The sugars attach by a chemical reaction and the sugar called fructose is known to be 10 times more reactive, and therefore more dangerous than our normal blood sugar (glucose).

Since the 1970s we have been using increasing quantities of refined fructose (from high-fructose corn syrup). Its appealing sweetness, and ability to suppress the 'no longer hungry' receptor (ghrelin receptor) is driving excessive food intake.[6] Its ability to damage our fatty nutrients and lipid circulation is also driving waist-line obesity and its associated health problems.[4,7]

Checking for Damage in our Lipids

There is a 'simple to administer' commonly available blood test used to check for sugar damage. It is used to check the proteins in the blood of people who are diabetic or at risk of becoming diabetic. It tests for Glycated Hemoglobin (HbA1c) by counting the proportion of damaged molecules (per 1000) of Hemoglobin protein in the blood (mmol/mol).

Researchers looking at ways of testing for damage to lipids, have found that the sugar-damaged blood protein test (HbA1c), presents a very reasonable approximation of the state of sugar-damage in the blood lipids. Until there is a good general test for sugar-damage in blood lipids, this test (HbA1c) could be a sensible surrogate. This is a better way of assessing health than a simple cholesterol test (TBSC).

Improved sugar-damaged blood protein (HbA1c) scores in diabetic patients are accompanied by improvements in their lipid profiles. This could be very useful to anyone wanting to improve health outcomes by managing lifestyle and nutrition.

Clinical Consequences of Lowering Cholesterol

In 2008 Dr. Luca Mascitelli asked me to examine a paper by Xia et al.[8] It was very interesting to note that lowering cholesterol by as little as 10% (molecular in cell walls) in the pancreas (pancreatic beta-cells) prevented the release of insulin (cholesterol-mediated exocytosis).

This paper described a mechanism by which 'cholesterol lowering drugs' directly cause diabetes. It was known that in statin drug trials which looked at glucose (blood sugar) control there was poor blood-sugar control in the statin user groups. Since 2011 the U.S. government (FDA) required statin packaging to carry a warning about the risk of causing diabetes.[9]

Memories are made of this – Cholesterol

The healthy human brain may only be 5% of body weight, but it requires over 25% of the body's cholesterol. The nervous system uses huge quantities of cholesterol for insulation, protection and structure (myelin). F.W. Pfrieger et al have shown that the formation of the memory (synapses) is dependent on good supplies of cholesterol.[10] Dr. Duane Graveline has researched and written extensively on the huge impact of statins on brain function.[11]

Post-mortem studies show that depleted cholesterol levels in the cerebrospinal fluids are a key feature of dementias. It was also reported that behavioral changes and personality changes are associated with low levels of cerebrospinal cholesterol.

In another review paper on dementia, our associates commented extensively on the damage done by fructose and the depletion of cholesterol availability.[7] Low cholesterol levels in the nervous system are not conducive to good mental health.

Consequences of Lowering Cholesterol

Drug treatments which lower cholesterol are acknowledged to cause adverse side effects (ADRs) in at least 10% of statin users.[12] This figure may be as high as 30%.

Conservative estimates indicate that for at least 1% of patients the side effects are serious enough to be life threatening (e.g. rhabdomyolysis, dementia, behavioral disorders and violence).

Our review[13] found that cholesterol lowering therapies were implicated in:

- Damage to muscles (including the heart) and exercise intolerance.[14]
- Increased risk of dementias (impaired synaptogenesis and neuro-transmission).[15]
- Failure of myelin maintenance (multiple sclerosis risks).[16]
- Neuro-muscular problems, aches and pains (amyotrophic lateral sclerosis - ALS).[17]
- Diabetes (insulin release inhibited).[8]
- Poor maintenance of bones and joints.

- Suppression of protective skin secretions (Apo-B) and increased MRSA infection.[18]
- Raised incidence of cancers.[19]

Again - Why would anyone want to lower cholesterol?

The Vital Role of Cholesterol

In history, cholesterol became an important evolutionary player when simple cellular organisms began evolving into the complex eukaryotic cells that gave rise to the animals.

The complexity of animal cells would not be possible without all the membrane structures that define the components of our cells. The nucleus, the mitochondria, the cell walls, the Golgi apparatus, the endoplasmic reticulum— all parts of our cells are contained by bi-lipid membranes. These bi-lipid membranes are a double layer of molecules with a fatty middle (lipophilic) and a water-attracting outer layer (hydrophilic).

While these membranes are basically the wrappers, they are also very dynamic, functionally active structures. They support and wrap the cell's contents. They support lipid traffic into and out of the cell and its organelles (internal cell parts).

To do this they need to be flexible, strong and changeable. A molecule is needed to move around the cell membrane, organizing and changing the bi-lipid layers in support of all its cellular functions. Only one molecule is uniquely suitable for this role – we know it as cholesterol.[20]

Many of the personal accounts quoted by Dr. Graveline in this book and in his other statin books, arise from the realization that it is cholesterol-reducing statins which are responsible for the many adverse health outcomes reported.

Therefore it is a puzzle that even after this experience, some people still feel compelled to reduce their cholesterol levels. The problem is no one seems to question the food and drug companies' advertising campaigns, which relentlessly depict our hero 'Mr Cholesterol' as one of the bad guys!

Over the last 40 years, even our doctors have been convinced by this incessant propaganda campaign against cholesterol. There has never been a scientific study that has been able to demonstrate a causal link between cholesterol and heart disease. The reality is that cholesterol, in its natural form, cannot be harmful.[21]

This has not stopped the marketing divisions of the pharmaceutical and food industries from creating an amazingly powerful and valuable myth, about an infamous household dietary and medical obsession, 'Bad Cholesterol'.

This has led to the shunning of natural cholesterol-rich foods, like butter, full-fat cheese, whole milk and eggs, in favor of processed vegetable trans fats and even sugar-rich low-fat foods.[19]

With doctors convinced that cholesterol was the cause of heart attacks and strokes, we switched to statins and unnatural fats like margarines. The harmful effects of trans fats were exposed in the 1950s by Professor Fred Kummerow and most recently in his 2014 book, *Cholesterol is Not the Culprit: A Guide to Preventing Heart Disease.*

The result of these 'commercial myths' is that the word cholesterol frightens people away from eggs and milk and butter and cheese — long established as the most natural foods for creating and rearing healthy offspring.

There is no evil in a cholesterol molecule. Cholesterol is just an incredibly fortunate breakthrough in the evolution of our cellular membrane chemistry.[20]

Almost all the cholesterol in our bodies is found in the cell membranes. An average of 20% of all the molecules in these cellular membranes is cholesterol. Over the past decade there has been a large increase in research publications documenting the action of cholesterol-rich lipid rafts within these membranes. Lipid research now describes an amazingly busy schedule for our membrane-cholesterol molecules which support everything we do.

With the emergence of the cholesterol-rich lipid raft hypothesis, the role of cholesterol in membrane function has become a focus of new research into exocytosis and endocytosis. Exocytosis is the process by which a cell guides the contents of secretory vesicles out of the cell membrane as lipid wraps.

These lipid wraps (membrane-bound vesicles) contain soluble proteins and lipids destined for functions outside of the originating cell. Endocytosis is the process by which cells absorb these lipid wraps and the molecules they carry (such as proteins) from outside the cell by engulfing it within their cell membrane, amoeba fashion.[22]

Lipid rafts are very rich in cholesterol, which organizes the other biochemicals in support of a variety of trans-membrane functions vital to cell recognition and communication.[23] This cholesterol has been shown to strengthen and stabilize the functional areas of the cell membrane. The physical consequences of cholesterol enrichment on the strength and thickness of membrane lipid-rafts were modeled and demonstrated by de Meyer, *et al.*[24]

The mediation of lipid membrane form and function by cholesterol affects the ability of a cell to perform exocytosis and endocytosis. The current trend in cardiovascular medicine to promote cholesterol reduction has caused concern in other non-cardiovascular branches of medicine. A growing number of researchers have identified the effects of cholesterol depletion on exocytosis and endocytosis with adverse consequences for our health.

Cholesterol depletion occurs when cholesterol levels in the body have been artificially lowered too far, as through the use of statins — reductase inhibitors. The inhibition of cholesterol synthesis is associated with functional failure of cholesterol-rich lipid rafts in processes such as exocytosis and endocytosis.

Cholesterol-rich lipid rafts support the receptor used to capture (SNARE) the lipid particles required by the cell.[25] These lipid particles transport the specific larger proteins and fat-soluble molecules that cannot simply pass by random diffusion through the cell membrane. This is a highly organized and vital lipid transport system mediated by cholesterol.

The cholesterol in the cell membrane also protects the cells' contents from leakage and loss. This is important when the cell stores energy, ready for some activity like thought (neuron) or exercise (muscle cell). The process of creating energy in all cells is dependent upon what is called electrochemical gradients, the accumulation of sodium ions or protons on one side of the membrane compared to the other, by pumping action through specialized membrane pores.

All animal plasma membranes use sodium for this purpose (members of the plant community use protons.) If adenosine triphosphate (ATP) is the gasoline that fuels our cells, sodium electrochemical gradients are the basis of the process that makes the ATP. The accumulation of sodium ions is accompanied by a natural leakage rate.

The reason for the cholesterol-rich layer of lipids in these plasma membranes is to prevent this leakage. Haines proposed in 2001 that cholesterol is a key inhibitor of sodium ion leakage.[26] Low cholesterol or any process that artificially lowers membrane cholesterol below natural limits must interfere with ATP production.

Of particular interest is Haines' discussion of comparable roles for both coenzyme Q10 and dolichols. Haines maintains that dolichols are responsible for leakage control of lipid for lysosomes (our intracellular disposal units), and ubiquinone (CoQ10) serves as control for our mitochondrial sodium ion leakage. Since statin drugs inhibit the synthesis of all three of these lipids (cholesterol, dolichol and ubiquinone) by the mevalonate blockade common to all reductase inhibitors, the work of Haines and other biochemists serves to document the inevitability of both mitochondrial damage and energy loss associated with statin use.

Haines has also studied the evolution of this mechanism from single cell through multi-cellular organisms, finding that the use of cholesterol for the purpose of inhibiting sodium leakage appeared very early, and has persisted for billions of years as the mainstay of ATP synthesis, demonstrating the persistence of successful mechanisms.

You can imagine that in the case of neurons and nerves, all the electrical activity transmitted down the connecting axons requires an elaborate containment of impulse and defense against burn out (oxidation).[16] Our neurons and nerves have evolved a protective wrapping of myelin. This myelin is continuously maintained by specialist cells. Oligodendrocytes maintain the myelin wrapping for the neurons, and Schwann cells maintain the myelin sheathing for our nerves.

Myelin is made up of about 40% cholesterol molecules and cholesterol is a very good insulator and antioxidant. Such large quantities of cholesterol, required by the oligodendrocytes, are supplied to the brain as an LDL lipid wrap called apolipoprotein E. The detail of the association of cholesterol depletion with dementias is investigated in the book by Dr Henry Lorin, *Alzheimer's Solved.*[27]

Pfrieger's landmark publication in 2003 of the vital role of cholesterol in the formation and function of memory synapses, has been followed by one research report after another documenting the importance of cholesterol and the wide-ranging demand for cholesterol in so many of our vital bodily functions, including nerve, muscle and even our personality.[10]

When looking at cholesterol research, I asked the basic question: 'What happens if you lower cholesterol levels in all tissues and organs throughout the body?' In answer, a catalogue of serious problems became evident and was already investigated and described in the literature.

A review paper, *Cholesterol-lowering therapy and cell membranes. Stable plaque at the expense of unstable membranes?* that I co-authored with L. Mascitelli and M. Goldstein, is now regarded as seminal and has been widely cited in other works.[13]

A retrospective analysis of a five-year trial showed a 30% increase in the incidence of diabetes associated with a cholesterol reduction therapy. More recently Xia *et al* demonstrated a causal link between membrane cholesterol lowering and the impairment of insulin granule release.[8] The effect of statins on glucose levels is well documented in a retrospective analysis of the JUPITER trial. Ridker discusses the effects of statin therapy on incident diabetes, having presented data showing that statins significantly promote diabetes in 6 out of the 7 trials listed.[28] [31] Our internal insulin supply is facilitated by cholesterol.

The impairment of the exocytosis of myelin has been cited as an explanation of the reduced myelination of our glial cells and Schwann cells (a form of glial cell responsible for the myelination of nerve fibers) critical for neural maintenance[16]. The maintenance and repair of our neurons and nerves requires huge amounts of cholesterol.

Inconclusive results in the use of statins for the reduction of bone loss and statin-associated fracture have implications for both the osteocyte (bone cell) and osteoblast (bone formation) action in bone remodeling.[29] The function of osteocytes and osteoblasts are mediated by cholesterol-rich lipid rafts through exocytosis and endocytosis. Bone repair and maintenance cells need cholesterol to function.

The loss of exocytotic secretions of apolipoprotein B, our major lipoprotein cholesterol carrier (LDL), and its role in immunosuppression, has been cited with regard to invasive skin infection.[18] Cholesterol-lipid particles are a big part of our ability to control and stop infections.

The diminished exocytosis of neuromuscular junction (agrin, LRP4 and MuSK) enzyme secretions has implications for associated neuromuscular junction disease symptoms (ALS), similar to myasthenia gravis, observed in long term statin use.[30] This is another instance where low levels of cholesterol can cause neuro-muscular problems.

The neurological effects of cholesterol depletion can produce a wide range of mental conditions. Commonly, severe anger and irritability may occur in many statin users. But depression, violent behavior, homicidal behavior and suicide are also known to be associated with cholesterol depletion.[13]

As Dr. Graveline explains later, neural systems have significant vulnerability to cholesterol depletion through the reduction in the synaptic function, using lipoprotein neuro-transmitters. Another greater vulnerability may be due to the loss of myelination in the protection of neurons from damage.[16] The protection of our brains and the creation of our every thought requires significant amounts of cholesterol.

Cholesterol is not only the most common organic molecule in our brains, it is also distributed intimately throughout the entire body. Additionally, cholesterol is the precursor for a whole class of hormones known as the steroid hormones that are absolutely critical for life as we know it. Such hormones include estrogen, progesterone, testosterone, aldosterone, cortisol and calcitriol (vitamin D).

These hormones determine our sexuality, control the reproductive process, and regulate blood sugar levels and mineral metabolism. And beyond this, there is yet another class of cholesterol's steroid offspring without which our metabolic well-being might be in serious jeopardy: the production of bile acids. Bile makes it possible for us to emulsify fats and other nutrients. Without bile, we could not digest and absorb the fats in our diet and must slowly starve.

We must also note that HMG-CoA reductase, the key enzyme target for statin use, is found in the membrane walls of the endoplasmic reticulum and the mitochondrial wall. These cell membranes contain between 20% and 50% cholesterol molecules. Our membrane-cholesterol is the very biochemical essence of our existence. How could anyone contemplate getting rid of it? What is needed is a lowering of damage to lipids — caused by sugar.

The large amount of cholesterol required for both the formation and function of these basic structures argues strongly against the rationality of excessively liberal use of drugs such as statins that inhibit cholesterol synthesis.

Based upon a presentation to the European Conference
Weston A. Price Foundation, London 2014
Glyn Wainwright, MSc, MBCS, CITP, CEng
Independent Researcher, Leeds, England, U.K.

References for:
The Wonder of Cholesterol

1.   Weiss, A., Beloosesky, Y., Schmilovitz-Weiss, H., Grossman, E. & Boaz, M. Serum total cholesterol: A mortality predictor in elderly hospitalized patients. *Clin. Nutr. Edinb. Scotl.* **32**, 533–537 (2013).

2.   Mancini, M. & Stamler, J. Diet for preventing cardiovascular diseases: light from Ancel Keys, distinguished centenarian scientist. *Nutr Metab Cardiovasc Dis* **14**, 52–7 (2004).

3.   Yudkin, J. *Pure, White and Deadly: how sugar is killing us and what we can do to stop it.* (2012).

4.   Seneff, S., Wainwright, G. & Mascitelli, L. Is the metabolic syndrome caused by a high fructose, and relatively low fat, low cholesterol diet? *Arch. Med. Sci. AMS* **7**, (2011).

5.   Bierhaus, A., Hofmann, M. A., Ziegler, R. & Nawroth, P. P. AGEs and their interaction with AGE-receptors in vascular disease and diabetes mellitus. I. The AGE concept. *Cardiovasc Res* **37**, 586–600 (1998).

6.   Lindqvist, A., Baelemans, A. & Erlanson-Albertsson, C. Effects of sucrose, glucose and fructose on peripheral and central appetite signals. *Regul. Pept.* **150**, (2008).

7.   Seneff, S., Wainwright, G. & Mascitelli, L. Nutrition and Alzheimer's disease: the detrimental role of a high carbohydrate diet. *Eur. J. Intern. Med.* **22**, 134–140 (2011).

8.   Xia, F. *et al.* Inhibition of cholesterol biosynthesis impairs insulin secretion and voltage-gated calcium channel function in pancreatic beta-cells. *Endocrinology* **149**, 5136–45 (2008).

9.   FDA publication. FDA Expands Advice on STATIN RISKS. (2014).   at http://www.fda.gov/downloads/ForConsumers/ConsumerUpdates/UCM293705.pdf

10.   Pfrieger, F. W. Role of cholesterol in synapse formation and function. *Biochim Biophys Acta* **1610**, 271–80 (2003).

11.   Graveline, D. *Lipitor Thief of Memory*. (Duane Graveline MD MPH).

12.   Roger Vadon (Producer). BBC File on 4 Statins. (2008).

13.   G Wainwright, L Mascitelli & M Goldstein. Cholesterol-lowering therapy and cell membranes. Stable plaque at the expense of unstable membranes? *Arch. Med. Sci.* **5**, 289–295 (2009).

14.   Hall, J. B. *Principles of Critical Care - Rhabdomyolysis and Myoglobinuria*. (McGraw Hill 1992, 1992).

15. Mauch, D. H. *et al.* CNS synaptogenesis promoted by glia-derived cholesterol. *Science* **294,** 1354–7 (2001).

16. Klopfleisch, S. *et al.* Negative impact of statins on oligodendrocytes and myelin formation in vitro and in vivo. *J Neurosci* **28,** 13609–14 (2008).

17. Goldstein, M. R., Mascitelli, L. & Pezzetta, F. Dyslipidemia is a protective factor in amyotrophic lateral sclerosis. *Neurology* **71,** 956; author reply 956–7 (2008).

18. Goldstein, M. R., Mascitelli, L. & Pezzetta, F. Methicillin-resistant Staphylococcus aureus: a link to statin therapy? *Cleve Clin J Med* **75,** 328–9; author reply 329 (2008).

19. Kummerow, F. & Kummerow, J. *Cholesterol is Not the Culprit: A Guide to Preventing Heart Disease.* (Spacedoc Media LLC, 2014).

20. Brown, A. J. & Galea, A. M. Cholesterol as an evolutionary response to living ... [Evolution. 2010] - PubMed - NCBI. *Evol. 2010 Jul6472179-83* doi:10.1111/j.1558-5646.2010.01011.x

21. Uffe Ravnskov & McCully, K. S. Vulnerable Plaque Formation from Obstruction of Vasa Vasorum by Homocysteinylated and Oxidized Lipoprotein Aggregates Complexed with Microbial Remnants and LDL Autoantibodies. *Ann Clin Lab Sci Winter 2009 Vol 39 No 1 3-16* at http://www.annclinlabsci.org/content/39/1/3.full

22. The 2013 Nobel Prize in Physiology or Medicine - Press Release. http://www.nobelprize.org/nobel_prizes/medicine/laureates/2013/press.html

23. Ikonen, E. Cellular cholesterol trafficking and compartmentalization. *Nat Rev Mol Cell Biol* **9,** 125–38 (2008).

24. De Meyer, F. & Smit, B. Effect of cholesterol on the structure of a phospholipid bilayer. *Proc Natl Acad Sci U A* (2009). at http://view.ncbi.nlm.nih.gov/pubmed/19225105

25. Lang, T. SNARE proteins and 'membrane rafts'. *J Physiol* **585,** 693–8 (2007).

26. Haines, T. H. Do sterols reduce proton and sodium leaks through lipid bilayers? *Prog Lipid Res* **40,** 299–324 (2001).

27. Lorin, H. *Alzheimer's Solved.* (BookSurge Publishing, 2006).

28. Ridker, P. M. Rosuvastatin to Prevent Vascular Events in Men and Women with Elevated C-Reactive Protein. *NEJM* 2195–2207 (2008). doi:10.1056/NEJMoa0807646

29. Sivas, F. Serum lipid profile: its relationship with osteoporotic vertebrae fractures and bone mineral density in Turkish postmenopausal women - Springer. *Rheumatol Int* **29,** 885–890 (2009).

30.   Kim, N. *et al.* Lrp4 is a receptor for Agrin and forms a complex with MuSK. *Cell* **135,** 334–42 (2008).

31. Cederberg, H. et al. Increased risk of diabetes with statin treatment is associated with impaired insulin sensitivity and insulin secretion: a 6 year follow-up study of the METSIM cohort. Diabetologia 58(5):1109-1117 (2015) doi:10.1007/s00125-015-3528-5.

The Wonder of Cholesterol.
Chapter Summary and Key Points.

- Our cells need cholesterol to function properly.

- High cholesterol is more often associated with good health and longevity.

- The rising obesity rates observed by the 1980s coincided with the widespread adoption of high-sugar, low-fat formulations in processed foods.

- Fats do not cause obesity or disease. It is the excess sugars which create abdominal obesity.

- Cholesterol levels are not measured, merely estimated from the quantity of very useful 'lipid droplets' circulating in your blood.

- LDL cholesterol does many jobs, like transporting vital fat soluble vitamins, lipids and proteins. Sugar-damaged LDL is not recognized by the organs that need these essential nutrients.

- It doesn't matter how high your total blood serum cholesterol is. What really counts is the damaged condition of the LDL lipids.

- As we age, excessive amounts of free sugars in the blood may eventually cause damage quicker than the body can repair it.

- HbA1c is a widely available blood test to check for sugar damage.

- Cholesterol-lowering drugs can cause diabetes.

- Cholesterol is vital for brain and nervous system functions.

- Behavioral changes, personality changes and dementias have all been associated with low levels of cholesterol.

- Cholesterol lowering drugs are known to cause adverse side effects in anywhere from 10% to 30% of patients.

Cholesterol Does Not Cause Heart Disease

By Dr. Duane Graveline

After extensive review of all available studies relating to the cholesterol lowering benefits of statin drugs, scientists reporting in the October 3rd, 2006 *Annals of Internal Medicine* pulled the rug out from under the government-sanctioned cholesterol levels for reducing cardiovascular disease. Their conclusion: "Current clinical evidence does not demonstrate that titrating lipid therapy to achieve proposed low LDL cholesterol levels is beneficial or safe."

What this means in plain English is that the theory of cholesterol causation for heart disease is incorrect. Cholesterol is not the culprit. What we have been taught since 1955 about the cause of atherosclerosis has been dead wrong.

To make matters even less understandable, several years earlier the government-funded National Cholesterol Education Program promoted new guidelines for the use of these drugs. It was recommended that individuals at high cardiovascular disease risk attain LDL levels < 100 mg/dL and individuals at very high cardiovascular risk attain LDL levels <70 mg/dL.

These are abnormally low levels of cholesterol, demanding high doses of powerful statin drugs if they are to be met. These artificially low levels of LDL cholesterol are grossly unnatural to the human body.

On July 13, 2004, the appointed experts published their recommendations for new cholesterol guidelines in the journal *Circulation of the American Heart Association*. The publication failed to disclose that six of the nine authors had direct financial ties to the makers of statin drugs. Those drugs included Pfizer's Lipitor, Bristol-Myers Squibb's Pravachol, Merck's Lovastatin, and AstraZeneca's Crestor.

These guidelines immediately boosted the sales of statins from fifteen billion per year when the report was released in 2004 to over twenty-two billion in 2005. And now we come to find out there is not a shred of scientific evidence to support that lowering cholesterol in this manner will reduce cardiovascular disease.

The October 3rd, 2006 review in the *Annals of Internal Medicine* tore this "solid science" to shreds, something that should have been done many years before. The review explains the deceitful manipulation of statistics and how not a single study proves that lowering LDL cholesterol to the very low levels recommended has any benefit in reducing cardiovascular disease, or that lowering your cholesterol one point from its present value has the slightest merit.

Simply put, this report was shocking to me. I had twenty-three years of active family practice. How do you think I felt about being so wrong in my prescribing habits by marching lockstep with my peers under the guidance of Big Pharma and the food industry, hand-in-hand with the American Medical Association and the American Heart Association?

I am still angry to think that nearly a quarter of my medical practice was based on a false concept about the origin of heart attacks and strokes. For me this was politics and medical science gone mad!

The bottom line is that there is no credible science, and there never was, that offered proof that lowering cholesterol levels to physiologically abnormal levels reduced cardiovascular risk. Creating a broad governmental public health program based on such rubbish was, and is, terribly wrong.

Why does this happen? It happens because many pharmaceutical-sponsored studies are published as if they are science. Mainstream media, heavily supported by pharmaceutical company advertising budgets, often tend to pass along the big Pharma sales pitch as is and the consumer all too frequently is left with the opinion that the sales pitch is based on solid science.

Now that tens of thousands of cases of side effects associated with the use of statin drugs have occurred, the same media, supported by millions of dollars in direct-to-consumer statin advertising, is understandably reluctant to support a wake-up to the American public.

For over forty years the cholesterol bandwagon with the enthusiastic support of both food and drug industries have guided clinical medicine. Throughout this time, physicians have written millions, if not billions, of prescriptions for whatever anti-cholesterol medication was in vogue at the time and have earnestly counseled their often skeptical patients about the evils of whole milk, eggs and butter.

Now more than forty years later, careful analysis of all available data including randomized trials, indicates that contrary to widespread opinion, cholesterol lowering does not appear to have a significant role in cardiovascular disease control.

Today there is a growing skepticism among practicing physicians for what Ancel Keys started back in the mid-fifties with his emphasis on cholesterol as the culprit for heart disease. The concept was easily sold at national levels and has guided health care for four decades.

This well-meaning Pied Piper and his flock of cholesterol followers has been like the Titanic — once in motion, difficult to stop. And has this growing doubt yet had any appreciable effects on statin sales? None that you would notice, and the focus on cholesterol reduction by the drug companies has never been stronger.

Show me a physician who is happy to admit he has been wrong for four decades; the same physicians who have been denying serious side effects from the powerful statin drugs. They are now awakening to the fact that they, like their disgruntled patients, may be victims themselves, duped by the incredible economic power of the food and drug industries to guide them along false paths in the name of profit.

These words are harsh but I have been saying these words for many years now and feel much like a broken record. I say them again and again for these words are true. Hardly a day goes by without additional support from the research community about the consequences of statin-associated mevalonate blockade. My words from over a decade ago remain as current today as the day they were written.

Cholesterol Does Not
Cause Heart Disease.
Chapter Summary and Key Points.

- The theory of cholesterol causation for heart disease is incorrect. Cholesterol is not the culprit.

- What we have been taught since 1955 about the cause of atherosclerosis has been dead wrong.

- New guidelines for LDL cholesterol are artificially low and grossly unnatural to the human body.

- Six of the nine authors of the new cholesterol guidelines had direct financial ties to the makers of statin drugs.

- There is no credible science that offers proof that lowering cholesterol levels to physiologically abnormal levels reduces cardiovascular risk.

Clinical Trials Challenge Cholesterol Causation

ENHANCE and IMPROVE-IT
Simvastatin plus Ezetimibe
(Zocor® plus Zetia® / Ezetrol®)

When the Effect of Ezetimibe Plus Simvastatin Alone on Atherosclerosis in the Carotid Artery (ENHANCE) trial results were announced in 2008, I said then that no study better proved the irrelevancy of cholesterol as a marker for cardiovascular risk.[1] In that study, the effectiveness of plain, generic, inexpensive simvastatin (Zocor) was compared with the more expensive Vytorin — consisting of the combination of simvastatin with ezetimibe (Zetia or Ezetrol.)

Zetia had already made millions, if not billions, by convincing the medical community that the addition of Zetia to gain an extra measure of cholesterol reduction was worth the extra cost. So enter gladiator Zetia into the arena with the result that although Vytorin resulted in much greater cholesterol reduction, the benefit in plaque status was no better than with Zocor alone

In this study, Zocor and Vytorin were pitted against the perceived atherosclerotic menace of familial hypercholesterolemia, using relative plaque thickness (IMT) of major blood vessels as their primary indicator of success.

For 24 months they had watched for progress and, at the end of the clinical trial, had been unable to see a significant difference evolving between the Vytorin and Zocor groups.

After behind-the-scenes deliberation about the possibility of changing endpoints, with rumors reaching all the way to the U.S. Congress, finally the lid was off and media feasting began. Even some of the most ardent supporters of cholesterol-lowering drugs attempted to distance themselves from the ENHANCE study with its dependence on direct observation of atherosclerotic plaque.

Vytorin is nothing but Zocor to which has been added Zetia, a non-statin cholesterol lowering drug acting on the gut absorption rather than on cholesterol synthesis. Those taking Vytorin in the study did get much lower LDL cholesterol levels, but it made no discernible difference. The implication is that LDL cholesterol lowering is not the key in atherosclerosis treatment or prevention.

Even the validity of the national cholesterol guidelines and the competence of those who draw up these guidelines is now called into serious question. This is what is causing great pain among these national and international leaders in the cholesterol war. This should not have happened, they think. They have said for years that LDL cholesterol must be lowered at all costs. This is what we all have been told for decades. Is something wrong here?

What is wrong is that these people with the anti-cholesterol philosophy are far better talkers than listeners. Had they been listening, they would have known that a growing number of people in the scientific community had been saying for years that cholesterol was irrelevant to the atherosclerotic process. Inflammation appeared to be the cause.

Cholesterol is nothing but an innocent bystander drawn into the plaques as part of the natural healing process. I have said before that labeling cholesterol as causative to atherosclerosis simply because it is there is roughly equivalent to blaming firefighters for fires because they are always there. For four decades physicians have been bombarded with this drivel. What has confused these statin advocates is the dual nature of statin drug effects on the human body.

Yes, statins are reductase inhibitors that reduce cholesterol synthesis through mevalonate pathway inhibition — unavoidably, statins also must decrease the synthesis of CoQ10, dolichols, selenoprotein and normal phosphorylation at the same time, but that is another story.

What we have learned only in the past decade is that statins are also powerful anti-inflammatory agents, exerting this effect via nuclear factor kappa B inhibition. Many now believe it is this anti-inflammatory effect of statins that is beneficial in atherosclerosis control, for atherosclerosis is an inflammatory disease.

The ENHANCE study simply helped to underline the irrelevance of cholesterol. This study showed rather dramatically that 80 mg of Zocor, however it is combined, is equivalent in effect and the addition of Zetia's cholesterol reduction did nothing more than sell Zetia.

The results of the IMProved Reduction of Outcomes: Vytorin Efficacy International Trial (IMPROVE-IT) — Ezetimibe Added to Statin Therapy after Acute Coronary Syndromes — published in June 2015 failed to provide evidence that the ezetimibe/simvastatin combination was significantly better than simvastatin alone.

Lowering of LDL cholesterol that extra amount through the use of ezetimibe gave no reduction in all-cause or cardiovascular mortality in the group taking simvastatin plus ezetimibe.

The results of this study, in my opinion, support my statement made 15 years ago that cholesterol is irrelevant to the effectiveness of statin drugs.

JUPITER
Rosuvastatin (Crestor®)

In January 2003, the Justification for the Use of statins in Prevention: an Intervention Trial Evaluating Rosuvastatin (Crestor) [JUPITER] investigators began to enroll 17,802 men and women with no evidence of cardiovascular disease and normal to low levels of low-density lipoprotein (LDL) cholesterol into a controversial trial.[2]

The participants in the trial had no evidence of heart disease but did have high levels of C-reactive protein (CRP). This trial was to test whether subjects with enhanced inflammatory responses (high CRP level) might benefit from statin therapy.

At study entry, none were considered candidates for statin therapy by the existing criteria. However, all trial participants had levels of the inflammatory bio-marker, high-sensitivity C-reactive protein (hs-CRP) equal to or greater than 2 mg/L, putting them at substantial risk for future cardiovascular disease.

These final selectees were divided into two groups. The test group received a mid-range dose of the commonly used statin, Crestor. The control group took a placebo. After 19 months the ethics committee ordered the test be stopped because of excessive numbers of heart attacks and strokes appearing in the control (placebo) group.

Because this study was considered potentially controversial from the very beginning, special pains were taken that the methodology be clear cut and unassailable.

The results of this study clearly indicated that cholesterol levels no longer should be considered a reliable risk marker for cardiovascular diseases and that statin drugs provided benefits for cardiovascular disease by an anti-inflammatory and immunomodulatory process having no relationship to cholesterol reduction.

Dr. Paul Ridker of Brigham and Women's Hospital directed the study and was deeply involved with this inflammatory biomarker. Dr. Ridker is listed as a co-inventor of this technique on patents held by Brigham and Women's Hospital. These relate to the use of inflammatory biomarkers in cardiovascular disease.

I will point out here that the use of the C-reactive protein test is far from new. As an intern at Walter Reed Hospital in 1955, I well remember ordering the CRP test as a non-specific test for inflammation. Because of its non-specificity it had limited usefulness. The high-sensitivity CRP (hs-CRP) version refers to improvements in sensitivity made since then. The hs-CRP test is thought by some to be a useful risk indicator of possible future cardiac events.

It was also about the time of this trial that the first grumblings about cholesterol causation came out. By then all of us, doctors and patients alike, had received three decades of intense brainwashing by the FDA, the drug companies and national medical organizations about the evils of cholesterol.

Hardly anyone in our country had any doubt about cholesterol culpability in cardiovascular disease. But, thankfully, there were a few leaders.

Kilmer McCully steadfastly refused to accept that something as natural and universal in our bodies as cholesterol could be the monster the drug companies were saying. As far as he was concerned, homocysteine accounted for some 40% of atherosclerosis and trans fats, oxycholesterol and smoking accounted for most of the others.

Uffe Ravnskov kept pointing out that if cholesterol caused heart attacks, how is it that most heart attacks were seen in patients with normal cholesterol. Clearly it made no sense to him and his book, *The Cholesterol Myths*, really opened my eyes.

Additionally, longitudinal studies with statin drugs were showing strange improvements in cardiovascular status regardless of which direction cholesterol values went. As long as the patient was on a statin they improved regardless of whether the cholesterol rose or fell. And the majority of acute heart attacks still happened in patients with normal and even low cholesterol. What was going on?

Unknown to the drug companies, one of the side effects of blocking the mevalonate pathway was inhibition of the critical transcriptase, nuclear factor kappa-B (NF-κB). In terms of cellular physiology, nothing happens in the areas of inflammation and immunodefense without NF-κB involvement. Today there is hardly a clinical physician who really understands this but to the medical researchers and the sharp minds in the drug companies, it changed everything. Atherosclerosis prevention became a new ball game, one that did not involve cholesterol. What were the national strategists for creating drugs in our society to do?

It was about this time that I made a prediction in my writings that the drug companies, despite their past three decades of self-serving, foul mouthing of cholesterol, were going to slide cholesterol out and slip inflammation in as a new cause of atherosclerosis, so deftly that they would not miss even one statin sale.

Do you suppose these companies were all that interested in the work of Doctor Ridker on inflammation? Short answer – yes. Now we are entering into the transitional phase of replacing cholesterol with inflammation. You may have already seen growing interest in your doctor's offices in doing your CRP test. Presently only hs-CRP has the specificity and sensitivity needed, but more markers will come along.

Many doctors are now wondering why they are using cholesterol-lowering doses of statins when cholesterol appears increasingly irrelevant to atherosclerosis. New dosing criteria have to be worked out. Already, forward thinking doctors are cutting the statin doses in an effort to get the desired anti-inflammatory effect without seriously interfering with mevalonate pathway function, the cause of many adverse reactions.

This will be tough going since the statin benefit is based upon mevalonate pathway inhibition of NF-κB. Much remains to be done, but it will be done. Cholesterol is out and inflammation is in.

In the JUPITER trial, statin treatment of apparently healthy individuals with elevated highly sensitive C-reactive protein (hs-CRP) and low LDL cholesterol resulted in similar and significant reductions in cardiovascular disease (CVD) risk for both women and men. Benefits appeared even greater in women despite their somewhat older age and higher levels of cardiovascular risk factors.

Primary prevention of risk reductions of CVD in women by one-third were reported, similar to prior results seen in men and in secondary prevention in women. Women in JUPITER appeared to have somewhat greater effectiveness in reduction of unstable angina, with men having a greater reduction in stroke incidence.

It needs emphasis that in the previous decade of clinical studies on the use of statins, most of them funded by the drug companies, no benefit had been documented for women and the elderly. We had begun to accept that the only group demonstrating significant statin benefit was middle-aged men. Now for the first time we found that women and the elderly of both sexes showed some benefit from use of a statin.

I must add here that physiology being what it is, what is true for men should be very similar for women as well and age should not make that much of a difference. So in this respect, the findings from JUPITER fit my "common sense" requirements much better.

Additionally there probably has never been a more closely controlled study from the viewpoint of methodology and data handling. Ridker and associates had designed a study that few could challenge successfully, although many have tried.

The JUPITER findings demonstrated for the first time the cardiovascular benefit from statin therapy for primary prevention in men or women selected for treatment on the basis of an elevated hs-CRP level, independent of their cholesterol. This highly sensitive C-reactive protein test has now been shown to identify asymptomatic women and men who are at increased risk of CVD events independently of their LDL cholesterol.

As I have written and as Ravnskov and McCully predicted much earlier, cholesterol is irrelevant to atherosclerosis. Statin drugs not only reduce cholesterol, for which they were originally created, but they also are powerful anti-inflammatory agents because of their ability to block the mevalonate pathway.

Not only is this the key to cholesterol synthesis, it leads also to reduction of CoQ10, dolichols and NF-κB, the transcriptase critical to inflammation suppression. The JUPITER study appears to have dramatically brought this into public focus and is clearly pointing the direction of statin treatment in the immediate future.

The new target is now elevated CRP and it is not only a far larger group but it is apt to be a younger group. Autopsies on casualties from the wars in Korea and Vietnam had documented the frequency of inflammatory lesions in young men with low and very low cholesterol levels that so mystified young doctors like myself.

We can expect wider screening and continued promotion of statins, but there will be one other major change — doctors will be less and less likely to be dosing statins at cholesterol-lowering levels. An individual's cholesterol levels are irrelevant and doses appropriate for inflammation have to be determined, or entirely new anti-inflammatory drugs have to be developed; drugs that somehow influence that NF-κB mechanism and our inflammatory and immune systems without interfering with the metabolism of CoQ10, dolichols and other biochemicals so critical to body function.

CETP Cholesterol Drug Fails
The ACCELERATE Study

On October 12th 2015, drug company Eli Lilly said it was halting a 12,000-patient study of its drug, evacetrapib, an oral cholesterol-lowering medication.[3]

In earlier studies, the treatment cut "bad" LDL cholesterol by 30 to 35 percent and doubled the levels of "good" HDL cholesterol. But the influence on cholesterol levels did not ultimately improve patients' health, dashing hopes for this approach to treating heart disease.

CETP (cholesteryl ester transfer protein) inhibitors suppress the process, whereby HDL cholesterol is transferred to LDL and VLDL (very-low-density lipoprotein). This causes a drop in serum LDL and VLDL and a consequent rise in HDL.

This improvement in lipid profiles, it was believed, would be of great benefit in reducing the risk of cardiovascular disease. But so far, this has not happened. Lower LDL and higher HDL have been of no benefit to the patients in the clinical trials.

In 2006, trials of Pfizer's CETP inhibitor, torcetrapib, were halted. Not only was no clinical benefit observed, but patients taking torcetrapib along with atorvastatin (Lipitor) had a 60% higher rate of death compared to those taking atorvastatin alone.

Hoffman - La Roche's CETP inhibitor, dalcetrapib, also raised HDL levels. But development of this drug was halted in 2012, "due to a lack of clinically meaningful efficacy."

As long as pharmaceutical researchers remain dedicated to cholesterol causality, I believe they will only find disappointment.

PCSK9 Inhibitors:
Injectable Cholesterol Reducers

In 2015, the U.S. Food and Drug Administration (FDA) approved the first two drugs of a new class of cholesterol-reducing agents known as PCSK9 inhibitors.

Proprotein convertase subtilisin/kexin type 9 (PCSK9) is a naturally occurring protein in humans that binds to the receptors for low-density lipoprotein (LDL) cholesterol in the liver. By inhibiting PCSK9, more LDL receptors are made available to attach to the LDL particles, thus reducing the amount of serum LDL cholesterol circulating in the body.

Although PCSK9 inhibitors are not statins, they are designed to be used in conjunction with statins for those patients that do not experience the expected drop in LDL cholesterol from statins alone.

They are also intended as an alternative method for reducing LDL cholesterol for the statin intolerant. Many of those that start a course of statins have to stop taking them due to muscle pain and weakness alone.

The first two PCSK9 inhibitors to be approved — Sanofi/Regeneron's alirocumab (Praluent) and Amgen's evolocumab (Repatha) — looked to have future competition with Pfizer's bococizumab. However, after reviewing data from large, late stage clinical trials, Pfizer announced on November 1, 2016 "the discontinuation of the global clinical development program for bococizumab," stating that, "bococizumab is not likely to provide value to patients, physicians, or shareholders." [4]

Approval for the marketing of alirocumab and evolocumab was granted only on the basis of LDL cholesterol reduction (which PCSK9 inhibitors do extremely well). At the time of approval, there was no evidence presented of any long term survivability or cardiovascular benefit for either of these biopharmaceutical drugs

Clinical trials to determine whether these drugs prevent either heart attacks or early death from cardiovascular disease are ongoing at this time.

So approval for these PCSK9 drugs was granted with no proven health benefit, an unknown long-term side effect profile, and at an annual cost more than 50 times higher than a generic statin. [5]

It is shocking to me that a drug could obtain approval based only upon treating a number, particularly when so many studies have shown that higher cholesterol equates to lower all-cause mortality.

Surely there should have been clinical trials showing actual benefit to those taking these drugs before releasing them for widespread use. How many of these early adopters realize that rather than taking a proven safe and effective drug that can extend their lives, they are part of an experiment with an uncertain outcome.

The results of the ongoing trials will be reviewed with much interest. As PCSK9 inhibitors work in an entirely different way than statins, there is no mevalonate blockade. So CoQ10, dolichols and selenoproteins, unlike with statins, will not be affected. This would suggest an improved side effect profile is possible.

However, there will be no anti-inflammatory benefit that is seen with statins and the same problems associated with artificially lowered cholesterol can be expected.

One of the negative effects of lowering cholesterol is cognitive issues. As we know, the healthy human brain is just 5% of body weight but contains over 25% of the body's cholesterol.

Remember also that cholesterol is an essential part of cell membranes, keeping them fluid and maintaining their structural integrity.

Cholesterol is also critical for the production by the body of steroid hormones like those responsible for regulating blood sugar levels, maintaining normal blood pressure levels and production of the sex hormones.

To create vitamin D from sunlight requires cholesterol and the body's ability to make bile acids to digest fats also relies on cholesterol.

I fear that all the drug companies are going to do with PCSK9 inhibitors, besides make money, is create incredible numbers of cognitive disorders of all kinds.

Neurocognitive problems, such as mental confusion or trouble paying attention, have already been noted to be present in some of the study participants receiving PCSK9 inhibitors.[6]

The PCSK9 monoclonal antibodies cut LDL cholesterol levels by an average of roughly 60% compared with placebo or standard therapy.[7]

Whatever our median serum cholesterol level has been during the time period 2004-2012 of our statin era, nearly 10,000 cases of transient global amnesia or severe memory loss have been reported to MedWatch during that time (4,809 cases of transient global amnesia and 4,235 cases of severe memory deficit).[8]

Imagine the impact on this marker when the median level of serum cholesterol approaches 50, the expected target level of LDL cholesterol, when this new class of drug is used along with statins.

In the original clinical trials for alirocumab, neurocognitive disorders were seen in those taking the drug compared to placebo.[9] These neurocognitive disorders included amnesia, memory impairment and confusional state — just what is seen with the use of statins.

So if you have two drugs, both independently capable of producing the same side effects, imagine what happens when you combine them. I cannot think of any act more guaranteed to cause neurocognitive chaos.

References for:
Clinical Trials Challenge Cholesterol Causation

1. http://www.nejm.org/doi/full/10.1056/NEJMoa0800742

2. http://www.nejm.org/doi/pdf/10.1056/NEJMoa0807646

3.https://investor.lilly.com/releasedetail.cfm?ReleaseID=936130

4. http://www.pfizer.com/news/press-release/press-release-detail/pfizer_discontinues_global_development_of_bococizumab_its_i nvestigational_pcsk9_inhibitor

5. http://www.msn.com/en-us/news/us/fda-approves-new-cholesterol-drug-at-dollar14600-a-year/ar-AAdsOdi

6. http://www.health.harvard.edu/blog/pcsk9-inhibitors-a-major-advance-in-cholesterol-lowering-drug-therapy-201503157801

7.http://www.medpagetoday.com/Endocrinology/GeneralEndocrinology/50546

8. FAERS Statin Review https://www.spacedoc.com/articles/faers-statin-review

9. http://www.nejm.org/doi/pdf/10.1056/NEJMoa1501031

Clinical Trials Challenge
Cholesterol Causation
Chapter Summary and Key Points.

- Contrary to widespread opinion, cholesterol lowering does not appear to have a significant role in cardiovascular disease control.

- In the ENHANCE study, those taking Vytorin did get much lower LDL cholesterol levels, but it made no discernible difference.

- LDL cholesterol lowering is not the key in atherosclerosis treatment or prevention.

- Cholesterol is nothing but an innocent bystander drawn into the plaques as part of the natural healing process.

- We have learned in the past decade that statins are also powerful anti-inflammatory agents.

- Many now believe it is the anti-inflammatory effect of statins that is beneficial in atherosclerosis control.

- Forward thinking doctors are cutting the statin doses in an effort to get the desired anti-inflammatory effect without seriously interfering with mevalonate pathway function, the cause of many adverse reactions.

- The JUPITER findings demonstrated for the first time the cardiovascular benefit from statin therapy on the basis of an elevated hs-CRP level, independent of cholesterol.

- CETP (cholesteryl ester transfer protein) inhibitors cause a drop in serum LDL and VLDL and a consequent rise in HDL.

- Lower LDL and higher HDL have been of no benefit to the patients in clinical trials.

- As long as pharmaceutical researchers remain dedicated to cholesterol causality, I believe they will find only disappointment.

- A new class of cholesterol reducing agents known as PCSK9 inhibitors came onto the market in 2015.

- Although PCSK9 inhibitors are not statins, they are designed to be taken with statins or alone for the statin intolerant.

- At the time of approval of the first PCSK9 drugs, there was no evidence presented of any long term survivability or cardiovascular benefit.

- In early clinical trials of a PCSK9 inhibitor, amnesia, memory impairment and confusional state were observed.

Mechanism of Statin Drug Benefit

During my past fifteen years of research on statins, my focus has been on the side effects of this class of drugs, specifically the impact of statin use on cognitive function, emotion and personality and the often permanent impact on muscles and nerves in the form of myopathy, neuropathy and ALS-like reactions.

Those unacquainted with the full range of my studies would quite naturally assume I am antagonistic to the use of statins, yet nothing could be further from the truth. For many years now I have supported the idea of statin use for high risk people and if it were me who suddenly became high risk, I would strongly urge my doctor to put me on a low-dose statin, but at a much lower dose than I was prescribed that led to my episodes with transient global amnesia.

Statins work to reduce cardiovascular risk, but the benefit they demonstrate has no relationship to cholesterol reduction; it is seemingly due to their powerful anti-inflammatory effect. Cholesterol reduction, the mantra for four decades, is irrelevant. During this time the scientific community has discovered the critical importance of cholesterol to body function, not only for the brain, but also for many vital cellular processes.

Instead of being public health's greatest enemy, as we have been brainwashed to believe these past forty years, cholesterol is probably the most important biochemical in the body. Not only is the cognitive function of our brains absolutely dependent upon ample supplies of cholesterol, but cholesterol is the reservoir from which many of our most important hormones such as estrogen, testosterone and cortisone are derived.

Additionally, every cell in the body is dependent upon cholesterol for myriads of vital cellular processes such as lipid rafting, exocytosis and endocytosis, most of which have only been delineated within the past few years, long after statins were first marketed. Why then the use of heavy doses of statin drugs to reduce this vital substance?

My war is not against the statins. Rather, it is against the use of these powerful reductase inhibitors to block cholesterol synthesis when, in the opinion of myself and a rapidly growing body of others, cholesterol levels have nothing to do with the development of atherosclerosis.

In the process of reducing cholesterol to lower and lower levels, we have managed to create varying degrees of mevalonate pathway blockade. It is this blockade of cholesterol, dolichol, CoQ10, selenoprotein, Rho (proteins) and normal phosphorylation that has caused the flood of reports of adverse effects from statins.

The blockade of cholesterol is the cause of most of the reports of cognitive dysfunction, but it is the CoQ10 and dolichol inhibition that is responsible for most of the other adverse effects of emotional and behavioral disorders and myopathies, neuropathies and atypical ALS.

The primary mechanism of action of statin drugs in cardiovascular disease control appears to be that of thromboxane inhibition, although much more study remains to be done.

Thromboxane means nothing to most of us, yet we all are very familiar with its effect. Anyone who has noticed a tendency for black and blue marks to appear much more easily while on aspirin knows a bit about thromboxane. So do those people taking a small dose of aspirin for heart attack or stroke control with the understanding that it will lower the likelihood of clot formation. This is another attribute of thromboxane. Triggered by blood platelets, thromboxane contributes to platelet aggregation and clot formation.

Aspirin acts by inhibiting the ability of platelets to stimulate the formation of thromboxane from arachidonic acid, reducing the risk of clotting. Low-dose, long-term aspirin use irreversibly blocks the formation of thromboxane by platelets, producing an anti-coagulant effect making aspirin useful for reducing the incidence of heart attacks.

In a landmark study, 112 individuals already on aspirin were given Zocor 40 mg daily with a close follow-up of selected inflammatory and coagulation markers. Zocor decreased serum thromboxane by 20 percent (from 1.32 to 1.06 ng/ml). Zocor decreased hs-CRP (high sensitivity C-reactive protein) very substantially from 2.06 to 1.39 inflammatory units. Zocor additionally decreased arachidonic acid levels from 9.6 to 5.4 units.[1]

Originally, in the early days of statin therapy, some were quick to come up with the name "super aspirin" for this new class of drugs. This study gives solid justification for this title although for marketing purposes the drug companies were not supportive of the somewhat demeaning "super aspirin" title. The primary effects of statins on platelet aggregation and clotting in this study were precisely those of aspirin. The only difference is in strength of effect. Three months of aspirin pretreatment produced the usually expected changes in thromboxane, hs-CRP and arachidonic acid, but the addition of statins substantially enhanced these effects.

The endothelium is the thin layer of cells that lines the interior surface of blood vessels, forming an interface between circulating blood and the rest of the blood vessel wall. These endothelial cells line the entire circulatory system. They are a variant form of our skin; a modification of our simple squamous epithelium.

Think of a tiny spot of damage, a divot in an otherwise featureless plain. It is in these endothelial cells that arachidonic acid, along with its precursors, are now suddenly and directly exposed to the blood stream and all its contents. This is where platelets come in to action. This is their entire purpose in life, to seek out these defects in the blood vessel walls.

Thromboxane-A synthase, an enzyme found in platelets, on sensing the presence of arachidonic acid, immediately begins the conversion of it into thromboxane. This powerful thrombotic agent also causes constriction of the blood vessels — stopping any further blood leakage — as well as facilitating platelet aggregation to bring in additional thrombotic resources.

Without further tweaking of the thrombosis/anti-thrombosis system, a thrombotic crisis could occur — a complete shutdown of circulation to the area with gangrene a possible consequence. This is where a substance known as prostacyclin comes into action.

Predictably, prostacyclin is produced in damaged endothelial cells by the action of a specific enzyme. The role of prostacyclin is primarily to inhibit formation of the platelet aggregation critical to hemostasis (stoppage of bleeding or blood flow). On one hand the platelet mechanism is trying desperately to cut down on blood flow through platelet aggregation while the endothelial-based prostacyclin mechanism is trying just as desperately to make certain that excess hemostasis is avoided.

Similarly, the vasoconstriction (narrowing of the blood vessels) of the platelet mechanism is offset by prostacyclin's vasodilation (widening of the blood vessels). Take heart from the fact that despite the past fifty years of research this subject remains an extraordinarily complex mechanism to everyone.

Despite there being much to learn about the various mechanisms involved, aspirin has continued to be widely endorsed by the medical community. Rarely do we find a drug so economical, effective and relatively safe. Numerous studies have shown that low dose aspirin taken daily is able to inhibit a large proportion of thromboxane, with prostacyclin synthesis being little affected.

In its manual *Aspirin in Heart Attack and Stroke Prevention*, the American Heart Association (AHA) recommends aspirin use for patients who've had a myocardial infarction (heart attack), unstable angina, ischemic stroke (caused by blood clot) or transient ischemic attacks (TIAs or "mini-strokes") if not contraindicated. The AHA manual states: "This recommendation is based on sound evidence from clinical trials showing that aspirin helps prevent the recurrence of such events as heart attack, hospitalization for recurrent angina, second strokes, etc. — secondary prevention. Studies show aspirin also helps prevent these events from occurring in people at high risk — primary prevention." In recent years many have challenged this recommendation, but for the overwhelming majority of practicing physicians, the message continues to serve.

The effect of non-steroidal anti-inflammatory drugs on platelet function and general topic of hemostasis is exemplified by Al Schafer's publication in the *Journal of Clinical Pharmacology*[2], titled "Aspirin and non-aspirin non-steroidal anti-inflammatory drugs (NSAIDs) inhibit platelet cyclooxygenase, thereby blocking the formation of thromboxane A2."

These drugs produce a systemic bleeding tendency by impairing thromboxane-dependent platelet aggregation and consequently prolonging the bleeding time. Aspirin exerts these effects by irreversibly blocking cyclooxygenase. Therefore, its actions persist for the circulating lifetime of the platelet. Non-aspirin NSAIDs inhibit cyclooxygenase reversibly, therefore the duration of their action depends on specific drug dose, serum level, and half-life. The only significant clinical difference is that one must stop taking aspirin for at least seven days before planned surgery. The usual platelet life span is seven to eight days, so this allows time for normal platelets to take over the job of stasis.

One wonders about the effect of chronic anti-coagulation through the use of aspirin and NSAIDs on prostacyclin production. The natural effect of prostacyclin is vasodilation and inhibition of platelet aggregation. Its production is inhibited indirectly by NSAIDs, which inhibit the cyclooxygenases enzymes COX1 and COX2. These convert arachidonic acid to prostaglandin H2 (PGH$_2$), the immediate precursor of prostacyclin.

Since thromboxane, also being downstream of COX enzymes, is being generated at the same time, one might think that the effect of NSAIDs would act to balance the two with neither thrombosis nor bleeding being in excess. However, prostacyclin concentrations recover much faster than thromboxane levels. Aspirin administration initially inhibits thromboxane and has little to no effect on prostacyclin, but eventually sufficient prostacyclin accumulates to prevent platelet aggregation.

It appears that the effectiveness of prostaglandins increases as they are regenerated. This is explained by understanding the basic difference in the two cells that produce thromboxane and prostacyclin. Since prostacyclin is primarily produced in a nucleated endothelial cell, the COX inhibition by NSAIDs can be overcome with time by increased COX gene activation and subsequent production of more COX enzymes to catalyze the formation of more prostacyclin.

In contrast, thromboxane is released primarily by blood platelets, which, having no nuclei, are unable to respond to NSAID COX inhibition with additional transcription of the COX gene because they lack DNA material necessary to perform such a task. This allows NSAIDs to result in prostacyclin dominance, thereby promoting vasodilation and anti-thrombosis.

In terms of the relative effectiveness of chronic administration of aspirin versus NSAIDs, one must infer that the use of aspirin must fall off somewhat because of gradual loss of the platelet aggregation factor, while with NSAIDs, the long-term use effects favor anti-thrombosis via prostacyclin effect. Both get the job done but with dissimilar mechanisms. Yes, this is terribly complex and if you are having trouble understanding these basic mechanisms you are not alone. There is no way to describe this process simply.

In an era where Big Pharma, the food industry and the medical community still could see no wrong with the broad scale use of statin drugs to lower our cholesterol "villain", Ora Shovman was introducing the concept in 2002 that atherosclerosis was a form of inflammation and was pointing out the possible role of autoimmune mechanisms in the development and progression of atherosclerotic plaque.[3] His assumptions were based upon histological evidence of the close relationship between the atherosclerosis plaque and such chronic inflammatory diseases as rheumatoid arthritis and cirrhosis. Additional support for the idea of atherosclerosis as an inflammatory reaction is the association of infection with atherosclerosis.

According to Shovman, the evolution of an atherosclerotic plaque involves an interaction between four major cell types: endothelial cells, smooth muscle cells, macrophages and lymphocytes. He saw that statins could be implicated in all of these elements of an inflammatory reaction.

Monocyte adhesion: He found statins to have an inhibitory effect on surface protein expression and adhesiveness between monocytes and the vascular wall.

Endothelial function: He found that statins altered the bioavailability of nitric oxide.

Macrophage activity: He found that statin treatment retarded plaque size growth and reduced macrophage accumulation.

Vascular smooth muscle cells: He found that statins impaired the process of smooth muscle cell proliferation and migration.

In conclusion, Shovman documented the basis for inflammation as the underlying process in atherosclerosis and supported the use of statins for their anti-inflammatory effect years before the JUPITER study.

It was Hilgendorff et al[4] who drew my attention to the effect of statins on inhibiting inflammation via blocking nuclear factor-*kappa* B (NF-κB) activation. In his paper "Statins differ in their ability to block NF-κB activation in human blood monocytes", his team demonstrated early on that the effect of statins went far beyond that of cholesterol reduction.

At the Justus Liebig University in Giessen, Germany, the results of their studies revealed that statins differ markedly in their effectiveness in preventing activation of NF-κB, a transcription factor involved in the activation of the early genes involved in inflammation.

Using six statins — atorvastatin (Lipitor®), cerivastatin (Baycol®), fluvastatin (Lescol®), lovastatin (Mevacor®), pravastatin (Pravachol®) and simvastatin (Zocor®) — his team tested for their ability to influence the induction of NF-κB in human monocytes during inflammation. All of the statins inhibited NF-κB binding activity in monocytes in a dose-dependent manner.

The inhibitory effect was due to reduced phosphorylation and was primarily dependent on the absence of mevalonate, the expected effect of reductase inhibitors — statins. While the effect appeared with all statins, there were marked differences in the degree of inhibition between the statins.

Of particular interest to me were their findings comparing degree of inflammation suppression with the range of statin dosages used. Even at the minimal dose of each statin there was already very substantial suppression of inflammation, in the range of 70 percent. Further dosage increases resulted in only minimal gains in inflammation suppression.

Supporting Hilgendorff's results, Bonnet and others compared the effects of 10-mg versus 80-mg Lipitor on hs-CRP levels, reporting that the lower dose gave 70 percent of the value of the higher dose.[5] In other words, one-eighth the dose gave nearly as much hs-CRP (high-sensitivity C-reactive protein) lowering. This type of study has been repeated many times with other statins giving similar results — the smaller dose having nearly as much effect as the higher dose on the reduction of inflammatory markers. The research evidence has allowed me to strengthen my belief that small doses might be able to trigger a satisfying anti-inflammatory effect without the risk of side effects known to result from mevalonate blockade.

The point here is that only minimal statin doses were necessary to produce most of the effect on inflammation suppression. I have for several years now believed that there should be studies to see whether statin sensitive people could tolerate very low dose statins (2 to 3mg of the newer, stronger statins). Then for the statin intolerant, a low dose of statin (in the hope of gaining anti-inflammatory benefit) would become an option, rather than stopping the drug entirely. The primary benefit of a statin without the dose dependent risk of severe side effects might then become an option. This has the potential to offer real benefits if inflammation, associated with excess free radical oxidation, is indeed the true cause of cardiovascular disease.

References for:
Mechanism of Statin Drug Benefit

1. Undas A. Int J Cardiol, Oct 28, 2010.
2. http://onlinelibrary.wiley.com/doi/10.1002/j.1552-4604.1995.tb04050.x/abstract
3. Anti-inflammatory and immunomodulatory properties of statins. Shovman O. Levy Y. Gilburd B. Shoenfeld Y. https://www.ncbi.nlm.nih.gov/pubmed/12018465
4. Hilgendorff. Internat J Clin Pharm and Therapeut, 41(9), 2003
5. Bonnet J. and others. Clin Ther, 30(12):2298-313, Dec.2008

Mechanism of Statin Drug Benefit
Chapter Summary and Key Points.

- I support the idea of statin use for high risk people, but at non-cholesterol lowering doses (low dose).

- Any cardiovascular risk benefit from statins has no relationship to cholesterol reduction.

- In addition to blockading cholesterol production, dolichols, CoQ10, selenoproteins and Rho are equally diminished by the effect of statins.

- Like aspirin, statins reduce the production of the blood clotting agent thromboxane.

- Blood levels of hs-CRP (high sensitivity C-reactive protein) — an inflammatory marker — are also reduced by statins.

- Aspirin has shown benefit in both primary and secondary prevention of heart attacks and strokes.

- Ora Shovman concluded that inflammation was the cause of atherosclerosis.

- Statins show cardiovascular benefits for their anti-inflammatory effect.

- Even at a very low dose of a statin, inflammation is suppressed substantially.

- Studies are needed to see whether statin sensitive people can tolerate low dose statins without the often debilitating side effects from higher doses.

Overview of
Statin Adverse Effects

When I was in medical practice, I was just like most of the doctors in the United States in that I considered cholesterol one of the greatest problems faced in public health. In response to the mandate from national leadership, I lectured to service clubs — and my sometimes skeptical patients — about the evils of whole milk, eggs and butter. I raised my family on no eggs, margarine instead of butter, and skim milk made from milk powder.

Such was my enthusiasm for cholesterol control, I must have written 10,000 prescriptions for whatever cholesterol-buster was available at the time. Therefore, during my astronaut physicals at Johnson Space Center back in 1999, when my NASA doctors prescribed Lipitor 10 mg daily for my cholesterol of 280, I took it without reservation.[1]

Six weeks later I had my first episode of transient global amnesia, and I suspected the possibility of an adverse reaction to my new and only medicine, Lipitor. But my doctors dismissed it. "Statin drugs don't do that," was the prevailing opinion. Nevertheless, I stopped the drug on my own, resolving to ask a few more questions.

The following year, when my NASA doctors strongly recommended I go back on Lipitor, and because my interviews during the year of some thirty doctors and pharmacists about possible cognitive side effects of statins proved consistently negative, I agreed to go back on Lipitor — but at half the previous dose: 5mg daily.

Eight weeks later I had my second attack of transient global amnesia. This time I was certain there was something about the statins we were not being told, but my doctors still felt it was an amazing coincidence.

Transient global amnesia is the abrupt onset, within seconds, of the complete inability to formulate new memory. This is usually associated with retrograde loss of memory for months, years or decades into your past. In my first episode the amnesia lasted for six hours with retrograde loss for some ten years into the past. As a result of this episode, I did not know my new wife, nor did I know my new home. I came to my senses in the emergency room listening to my wife tell me how her day and mine had gone. I was naturally amazed and quite anxious.

The following year, my episode of transient global amnesia lasted for twelve hours. During this episode I was a thirteen–year-old high school student with full recall for that particular day's assignments, teachers, books and classmates, but I laughed hysterically when they told me I was married with children and was a family doctor. I could not have doctored a mouse and knew nothing of marriage. I was thirteen years old!

All that the drug companies ever really told us about the mechanism of action of statins was that they were reductase inhibitors. Not believing that we were being told only half-truths that might have serious repercussions, doctors took this information at face value. After all, we were on the same team.

Had we but reviewed our dusty biochemical textbooks for just a few minutes, we would have learned the truth. This reductase step that was so interesting to drug company researchers just happened to be at the very beginning of the mevalonate pathway, responsible for the synthesis of not only cholesterol (our target at that time) but also such vital substances as CoQ10, dolichols and selenoproteins and even normal phosphorylation.

Every first-semester student of biochemistry knows you cannot do this without risk of very serious side effects. Cholesterol reduction was top priority, and with the promise of vast profits, the drug companies went ahead with their mevalonate blockers.

This was no mistake. Their researchers knew what the risks were but management ordered it done, regardless.

When Frank Pfrieger reported in *Science* magazine in 2001[2] on the extreme importance of brain cholesterol to memory, the reaction of the drug industry and FDA was, "no comment". Not a word was said about a side-effect of major importance linked to cholesterol reduction, or that of impaired cognition. Amnesia was just the tip of the iceberg in terms of peoples' reactions. Most reported confusion, disorientation and extreme forgetfulness, as well as dementia–like manifestations.

It seems that our brains are so dependent upon cholesterol for the formation and function of memory synapses that special cells in the brain — our glial cells — synthesize cholesterol as it is needed. Naturally this glial cell process was inhibited by statin drugs. We had an obvious culprit. Cognitive dysfunction represented a group of symptoms based upon excess cholesterol inhibition resulting from statin use. Most of the other problems we see represent collateral damage to these other participants in our mevalonate pathway — the CoQ10, dolichols, etc., substances critical for body function abruptly inhibited by statin use because of mevalonate blockade.

The full range of statin side effects goes far beyond cognitive dysfunction to include behavioral and emotional disorders, chronic nerve and muscle damage, and an ALS-like neuromuscular degenerative process as major categories of damage.

Thousands of statin users have been afflicted with peripheral neuropathies, with a tendency to be resistant to all traditional medical treatment. We have learned also that muscle damage cases are far more than the original drug company estimates of less than 2% — as high as 15% have been suggested.

Far more important than this incidence figure is the fact that according to Golomb, some 68% of these myopathies will become permanent and like the neuropathies prove to be remarkably resistant to all traditional forms of treatment.[3] The increased numbers of ALS-like cases seen in statin users world-wide was reported by Ralph Edwards in 2007.[4] At the time, he was the Director of the World Health Organization's VigiBase™ system in Uppsala, Sweden. As an international drug monitoring system, VigiBase can be considered as the counterpart of the U.S. Food and Drug Administration's MedWatch.

While searching for an answer as to why these effects of statins are permanent in so many people, I discovered the truly dark side of statins. They are hastening the natural process of mitochondrial mutations.

You may have been on one of the statins for a few months and noticed a few aches and pains, and that your memory is going a little awry. You may have mentioned this to your doctor and he or she tells you, "You have to expect this now you are getting older." This scenario replays again and again as new statin victims first encounter the premature aging effects of statins.

Yes, all of us undoubtedly are getting older and that handy repartee may get your doctor off the hook, but it is far more likely that your new symptoms have nothing to do with natural aging. Your failing memory, lack of stamina, unsteadiness and weakness are far more likely to be side effects of your statin drug. The strange thing about this is that your doctor has put his or her finger on the problem of premature aging without once suspecting the truth.

In the past few years we have learned much about the aging process and CoQ10 appears to be right in the middle of it. Few of us realize how vital CoQ10 really is. Years ago, in the early stages of my research on the side effects of statin drugs, I discovered the three primary functions of CoQ10 and I was impressed not only with how important this biochemical is but with the fact of how rapidly our ability to synthesize it plummets with aging.

By the time we reach fifty, we are almost completely dependent upon ingested CoQ10. The average diet contains very little CoQ10; the best sources being meat and fish, with the richest dietary sources being beef, chicken and pig hearts and to a lesser extent liver. Animal hearts are not consumed regularly by most people.

I soon discovered the special role of CoQ10 as an antioxidant to our mitochondria. We have dozens of natural antioxidants but only CoQ10, with a free radical quenching ability some 50 times greater than that of vitamin E, is bonded directly to our mitochondria, vital to both its structure and function. Without adequate stores of CoQ10 and lacking the repair mechanisms common to nuclear DNA, irreversible oxidative damage to mitochondrial DNA results from excessive build-up of superoxide and hydroxyl radicals.

We must remember that our mitochondria are in immediate contact with oxygen; front line warriors, so to speak, in the struggle to obtain life-giving oxygen without sustaining excessive oxidative damage. The inevitable result of excessive free radical accumulation is an increase in the rate of mitochondrial mutations.

The fact that we must repair thousands of mitochondrial DNA mutations daily in our bodies from the normal process of converting food into energy is not widely known. This daily load of oxidative damage is due to the excess energy of oxygen radicals released during normal metabolism.

Each one of these substitutions and deletions on DNA strands must first be identified, then excised and finally replaced with the correct form so that we continue to function. Our dolichols are vital to this process in that each step of our mitochondrial DNA correction requires a specific glycoprotein-derived enzyme. Dolichols orchestrate this entire process of glycoprotein synthesis and statins have long been known to inhibit dolichols.

But even more important is the critical importance of the powerful antioxidant role of CoQ10. Statins inhibit the functional availability of CoQ10 in complexes I and II of our mitochondria's energy producing sequence, causing suppression of CoQ10's normal role of reducing this daily oxidative load.

Some studies demonstrate as much as a 50% decrease in CoQ10 availability within a few weeks of starting statins. The end result here is a one-two punch wherein statins inhibit not only dolichols, corrupting our DNA damage correction, but CoQ10 as well, increasing our damage load.

Predictably the inevitable effect is increased mitochondrial DNA damage — considered by many authorities to be the mechanism of our aging process as well as that of many chronic diseases. Statins block the synthesis of CoQ10 and dolichols, thereby contributing directly to the premature common chronic ills of aging.

Since this involves normal physiologic processes, it is silent. By the time we become aware of it, it is already far too late and the damage has been done to those who are susceptible. This, in my judgment, is the truly dark side of statins.

References for:
Overview of Statin Adverse Effects.

1. Graveline, D. *Lipitor, Thief of Memory.* 2003
2. Pfrieger, F. Brain researcher discovers bright side of ill-famed molecule. Science, 9 November, 2001
3. Golomb, B.A., Evans, M.A. 2008. "Statin Adverse Effects: A Review of the Literature & Evidence for a Mitochondrial Mechanism." *American Journal of Cardiovascular Drugs.*March 2009
4. Edwards, R. ALS and statins. Drug Safety 2007;30(6):515-525.

Overview of Statin Adverse Effects
Chapter Summary and Key Points.

- I practiced medicine at a time when cholesterol was *Public Enemy Number One.*

- Six weeks after starting Lipitor, I had my first episode of transient global amnesia (TGA).

- A year later, after re-challenging with Lipitor, I had my second attack of TGA.

- The brain is dependent upon cholesterol for the formation and function of memory.

- The full range of statin side effects goes far beyond cognitive dysfunction to include behavioral and emotional disorders, chronic nerve and muscle damage and an ALS-like neuromuscular degenerative process.

- Statins speed up the natural process of mitochondrial mutations.

- Statins deplete CoQ10 and few realize how important CoQ10 is.

- By the time we reach fifty we are almost completely dependent upon a dietary intake of CoQ10.

- We must repair thousands of mitochondrial DNA mutations daily in our bodies from the normal process of converting food into energy

- CoQ10 has a powerful antioxidant role.

- Statins block the synthesis of CoQ10 and dolichols and contribute directly to the premature, common chronic ills of aging.

- The inevitable effect of lowered CoQ10 and dolichols by statins is increased mitochondrial DNA damage.

Statin Drugs, Side Effects Review

My first statin book, *Lipitor®, Thief of Memory,* was written after my two bouts of transient global amnesia (TGA) associated with the use of Lipitor® in the years 1999 - 2000. Predictably at that time, I was focused on cognitive dysfunction and Lipitor.

After my TGA episodes, I had been left knowing that my MRI was normal and even though several other statin users had shared my TGA experience, I was still concerned about the possibility of underlying organic disease.

For the first time, the work of Frank Pfrieger and others on the importance of cholesterol to brain function, gave the medical and scientific community the knowledge of glial cell synthesis of cholesterol and the absolute necessity of cholesterol for both the formation and function of memory.

Until that time nobody in the medical community seemed to understand how a statin drug could adversely affect cognitive function. Cholesterol in the blood must be carried about attached to lipoproteins so that the resulting molecule is much too large to pass the blood-brain barrier and is therefore unavailable to the brain. Abruptly I had my answer to my amnesia episodes.

Our brain cholesterol comes from specialized housekeeper cells in the brain — known as glial cells — whose task, among many others, is to produce cholesterol upon demand. Only in the presence of this cholesterol can memory function take place. Humans have evolved with this mechanism of brain function and cholesterol is absolutely vital to the process. The glial cells, our only source of brain cholesterol, are inhibited by statins just like every other cell in our bodies. Without sufficient availability of cholesterol, memory must falter. It is inevitable!

I finally had my mechanism for memory impairment and by now hundreds of emails were coming in to me from those now aware that statin drugs had the ability to seriously impair cognitive function. In just a few months I had 30 cases of transient global amnesia reported to me and Dr. Beatrice Golomb, director of the National Institutes of Health (NIH) funded statin study at the University of California, San Diego (UCSD) College of Medicine. Dr. Golomb invited me to co-author her paper for submission to the *Archives of Internal Medicine* to share this information with the medical community.

As a former United States Air Force (USAF) and civilian flight surgeon, I was particularly concerned that pilots and others on flying status were being permitted use of these statin drugs. What if I had been flying my plane when one of these amnesia episodes hit? You have no warning and in my first episode of TGA, I retrograded 10 years. In my second, 56 years. I was abruptly 13 years old for an amazing 12 hours. Obviously in my second experience, my flight training — like my marriage with children and my training as a doctor — had not yet taken place. To suddenly "awaken" in the cockpit of a strange, never-before-entered flying machine would have been an incredible experience, almost inevitably ending in death.

The medical community needed to have this information. You can imagine my reaction to learn that the *Archives of Internal Medicine* rejected the manuscript. Two months later we submitted this paper to the *Annals of Internal Medicine* and they rejected it as well. Both Dr. Golomb and I had abundant experience with submitting papers for publication.

It was a very well written paper disclosing a new reality, one that the "powers that be" controlling the peer review process were not ready to accept. Statins were simply too good. If anything, "they should be put in the drinking water" was the prevailing climate at that time. MDs did not want to hear of annoying side effects of their promising statins and the last thing the drug companies wanted to see was their golden goose tarnished.

Finally, in August of 2003, a team of researchers led by Dr. Wagstaff at Duke University managed to publish their paper titled, "*Statin-Associated Memory Loss: Analysis of 60 Case Reports and Review of the Literature*".[1] Published in *Pharmacotherapy* journal, the researchers searched MedWatch records for statin-associated memory loss. MedWatch is the U.S. Food and Drug Administration's formal electronic reporting system for post-marketing surveillance of new drugs in the United States. They found that: "about 50% of the patients noted cognitive adverse effects within 2 months of therapy".

Pharmacotherapy journal was sufficiently liberal to publish what should have been a headline-grabbing article. However, the readership of this journal is such that there was not the slightest impact on the prescribing habits of MDs, nor the slightest evidence of cognitive side-effect awareness. There was simply no discernable reaction from the community of clinicians who write the prescriptions for statins.

In 2007, I managed to acquire a copy of MedWatch raw data for Lipitor from the period 1998 through 2006, and using the same criteria as Dr. Wagstaff, I found 662 reports of TGA or comparable memory dysfunction.[2] On the basis of reported rates of TGA seen throughout the last year of my data (2006), I could project with reasonable validity that the total number of such reports received at the time (Oct. 2009) would easily exceed 1,000.

Far more important than that projection, and knowing that five more commonly used statins also have contributed their share of cognitive dysfunction during this same time period, is the fact that not one word of this observation had been officially reported by the FDA to the medical and scientific communities. The average prescribing physician was still completely unaware of the cognitive impact of statins.

Only on February 28th, 2012 did the FDA finally announce an update to the safety label for statins.[3] This update now includes *"cognitive side effects (memory loss, confusion, etc.)"* as known adverse events from statins. This official acknowledgement of cognitive side effects including memory loss came eight years after the first edition of *Lipitor®, Thief of Memory* was published, in which I thoroughly covered this side-effect potential of statins.

We must also remember that TGA is only the tip of the iceberg in that for every case of TGA reported, hundreds of cases of statin-associated confusion, disorientation and increased forgetfulness have occurred.

I have received many e-mails over the years from people on statins who have had cognitive loss episodes. Common examples have been while driving a car. The red light changes to green and they suddenly have no idea what to do next; momentarily they have forgotten how to operate the vehicle. Or as they get close to home, they recognize the places around them, but have no idea how to get to their own house, even though they may have done it hundreds or even thousands of times before.

Many cases of statin-associated cognitive impairment are misdiagnosed as Alzheimer's disease or other forms of dementia. Additionally, hundreds of short-term TGA's measured in minutes rather than hours almost undoubtedly have occurred during this time period, only to be completely missed unless an attentive observer was present to document it. The victim would be completely amnestic for this experience and therefore have no recall that it even occurred.

The classic definition for transient global amnesia is the abrupt inability to formulate new memory for a time period ranging from 2 to 24 hours. Any duration longer than 24 hours is increasingly likely to have an organic basis. No mention is generally made of the fact that there is no neurophysiologic reason why TGAs measured in minutes cannot occur. A TGA lasting for minutes would be impossible to detect by the victim and quite difficult even for a perceptive observer.

When a TGA victim is unobserved, only the passage of time as evident by the position of the sun in the sky or time passage as recorded by a time-piece (if one is available) might provoke a TGA victim to consider that a serious time loss had occurred.

So I had my explanation for cognitive dysfunction and *Lipitor*®, *Thief of Memory* is still the best background information book for those with primarily cognitive impairment. However, I soon became aware that much more was happening to statin users than cognitive dysfunction.

Statin drugs affect a single reductase step along the biochemical path of cholesterol synthesis. What does this really mean? From the very beginning, the Merck pharmaceutical company announced the fact that their statin worked by a mysterious process known as reductase inhibition. We physicians perhaps should have been more perceptive, for even a glance at the biochemical pathways would have told us something very worrisome was possible; but we trusted the drug companies. We were so pleased with this new statin, lovastatin (Mevacor), with its capacity to drastically lower cholesterol, we simply forgot to ask critical questions.

After 40 years of anti-cholesterol brainwashing we all agreed that cholesterol was our enemy and none of the many drugs we had used during that time really had much effect on cholesterol. Any drug that could almost guarantee to lower this biochemical by 40-50 points in a few weeks simply had to be good.

It was in this climate that I wrote my second book, *Statin Drugs Side Effects and the Misguided War on Cholesterol*, for our problems were far more than cognitive, and all statins were contributing to the rising tide of adverse reactions, not just Lipitor. This is when I learned what reductase inhibition really meant.

The reductase step, that all biochemists know as susceptible to blockade, was at the very beginning of the mevalonate pathway. This pathway to cholesterol synthesis is also shared by many extremely important biochemical substances, including CoQ10, dolichols, selenoproteins, normal phosphorylation, Rho (vital for cognition) and nuclear factor kappa B (NF-κB).

These are all extraordinarily vital to human function and to block this pathway — with statins — sufficiently to reduce cholesterol production, then synthesis of these other biochemicals must also be inhibited. It is not just possible, it is virtually guaranteed. One cannot reduce cholesterol by the use of statins without simultaneously blocking these other biochemicals sharing the mevalonate pathway.

This is much like the girding of a tree trunk — all the branches are inhibited, not just the cholesterol branch. This is the cause of most of the known side effects. The neuropathies, myopathies, rhabdomyolysis, emotional and behavioral disorders and even certain neuro-degenerative conditions such as ALS-like conditions are side effects based on mevalonate pathway inhibition. Even the one solid good that statins appear to do — the reduction of atherosclerosis risk — is probably a previously unsuspected side effect from the inhibition of nuclear factor kappa B (NF-κB), a powerful anti-inflammatory substance felt by most biochemists to be dependent upon the mevalonate pathway for synthesis. Cholesterol lowering has nothing to do with it.

The results of longitudinal studies had strongly indicated the presence of non-cholesterol factors. This was suggested from observations of a positive cardiovascular protective effect evident in many studies, even when cholesterol failed to respond to statins. In addition, new myocardial infarction cases (heart attacks) consistently showed that 50% had normal to low cholesterol values. These observations have made most objective researchers seek non-cholesterol factors such as inflammation as a major cause of atherosclerosis.

Trans fats, oxycholesterol, omega-3/6 imbalance, cigarette smoking and hidden chronic infections are well known triggers to inflammation. This is further supported by the more recent demonstration of a solid relationship between CRP (C-reactive protein) elevation — a measure of inflammation — and underlying cardiovascular risk.

My second book, *Statin Drugs Side Effects*, continues to be very relevant, and mevalonate blockade remains a major cause of side effects, but something new has now been added.

Then I began to ask questions, such as: "Why do the neuropathies, myopathies and other neurodegenerative conditions such as ALS often become permanent? If CoQ10 deficiency played such a major role in the etiology of these conditions, why is it that these conditions persisted despite vigorous attempts at restoration of CoQ10? What was causing this failure of response in so many cases?" These are fair questions, and a reasonable answer was long in coming, but finally it arrived. The answer was mitochondrial mutations.

This is when I discovered that although mevalonate inhibition of CoQ10 may have played a major role in causing the initial problem, the mitochondrial change it triggered had made the condition permanent. At that point, even an over-abundance of CoQ10 could not reverse the course. This made sense to me, and I soon found plenty of support from within the research community.

I knew I was on the right track with my third book, *The Statin Damage Crisis,* a vital information resource, especially valuable to those having permanent side effects from prior statin use. This is truly a crisis, for now we understand that to give statins without also giving CoQ10 is to invite disaster. Other countries such as Canada had specifically warned of this and strongly advised CoQ10 and even L-carnitine supplementation from the very beginning. The United States did not. This has been the cause of many thousands of cases of permanent damage and disability from statin use.

Few of us knew of Merck's request to the U.S. Patent Office back in 1990 to permit them the addition of CoQ10 to their new statin, lovastatin (brand name Mevacor®). If our vigilant media took special interest in this unusual request on the part of a drug company, I must have missed it. When Merck's patents were granted, they were promptly shelved and the company went on about the business of selling plain Mevacor.

Sadly it seems that doctors are no longer on the same side as the drug companies. Major pharmaceutical companies are beholden to their stockholders first. The health and well-being of the public seems much further down on the list — barely evident at times — and all statin makers have just played follow-the-leader.

Then in the era 2005-2007, news about cholesterol's possible irrelevance appeared. We could all eat eggs and butter again, we were told. Statins worked, we were gradually discovering, not by cholesterol reduction but by their powerful anti-inflammatory action.

Atherosclerosis was basically an inflammatory process starting first in the sub-endothelial region of the arteries and demonstrating the four major elements of inflammation: platelet activation, monocyte adhesion, macrophage attraction and smooth muscle migration, all inhibited by the novel anti-inflammatory action of statins.

Now the proper treatment began to involve the use of anti-inflammatory agents. Study after study proved this effect of statins. Aspirin has a very similar effect, justifying the use of the term super-aspirin, in vogue for a while, to describe the action of statins. However, the drug companies were quick to inform us that statins worked better than anything else we had for vascular inflammation and could be used successfully for almost anything having an inflammatory component such as auto-immune diseases and organ transplant rejection.

But they made certain to keep the waters muddy with respect to cholesterol. After four decades of brainwashing and almost two decades of use, what doctor seriously wanted to accept a new causation for atherosclerosis? How could you tell your patients you had been wrong all this time?

Our new cholesterol disease was rapidly disappearing. In its place was rising a new edifice to the role of inflammation. How best to handle this confusing fact from the viewpoint of the drug industry? Simply pretend it isn't happening. Keep the doctors focused on cholesterol as long as possible, for billions of dollars are at stake, and if we play our cards right we might slide cholesterol out and inflammation in and never miss a statin sale. As to the side effects of statins, we will pretend we do not hear about them.

References for:
Statin Drugs, Side Effects Review

1.http://onlinelibrary.wiley.com/wol1/doi/10.1592/phco.23.7.871.3272 0/abstract
2. https://www.spacedoc.com/articles/662-cases-memory-loss
3. http://www.fda.gov/Drugs/DrugSafety/ucm293101.htm

Statin Drugs, Side Effects Review
Chapter Summary and Key Points.

- My interest in the side effects of statin drugs began with my personal experience of two episodes of transient global amnesia (TGA) after taking Lipitor.

- Cholesterol is essential for brain and memory function.

- The cholesterol that the brain needs is produced in the brain itself by glial cells and reduced by statins as in the rest of the body.

- Without sufficient availability of cholesterol, memory must falter. It is inevitable!

- Both TGA episodes came on abruptly, temporarily blocking any memory of events stretching back decades.

- Four years after my first TGA, a paper was published: *"Sixty cases of transient global amnesia reported to FDA's MedWatch"*. I was not alone.

- Not until February 2012 did the FDA warn of *"cognitive side effects (memory loss, confusion, etc.)"* as known adverse events from statins.

- For every case of TGA reported, hundreds of cases of statin associated confusion, disorientation and increased forgetfulness have occurred.

- Many cases of statin associated cognitive impairment are misdiagnosed as Alzheimer's disease or other forms of dementia.

- I soon learned that statin problems were far more than just cognitive and all statins were involved.

- The pathway to cholesterol synthesis is also shared by important biochemical substances including CoQ10, dolichols and selenoproteins.

- The neuropathies, myopathies, rhabdomyolysis, emotional and behavioral disorders and ALS-like conditions are side effects based on mevalonate pathway inhibition by statins.

- Non-cholesterol factors such as inflammation are now implicated as a major cause of atherosclerosis.

- Trans fats, oxycholesterol, omega-3/6 imbalance, cigarette smoking and hidden chronic infections are well known inflammation triggers.

- I wondered why many of the side effects became permanent in some people and the answer was mitochondrial mutations.

- To give statins without also giving CoQ10 is to invite disaster.

- The "cholesterol disease" explanation for atherosclerosis is rapidly disappearing with the role of inflammation now in the spotlight.

Dolichols, Statins and Personality Change

Whether to be bound to a cell surface or destined to be secreted, proteins, those magic particles so important to our function and destiny, are synthesized within the membranes of the endoplasmic reticulum (ER), a tubular marvel of complexity within each of the body's cells.

It is within this microscopic structure that amino acids are linked together into a peptide, like a popcorn string. Some peptides will ultimately serve for cell identification so they may wander about our immune system without being challenged; others produce insulin because our blood sugar is rising or make us fall in love because of the attractive qualities of that person to us.

This class of proteins contains a signal as a recipe to guide the ER assembly of our necessary peptide, thereby matching our immediate needs.

This entire process is orchestrated by dolichols in the form of dolichol phosphate. In terms of chain of command, I cannot tell you who issues the command for a certain peptide, for that is beyond our understanding at this time, but the command once given is carried out by dolichol, the executive officer of this amazing process. We are dealing with a factory producing a substance under an administration process familiar to any production line facility.

In case you have not already suspected, this peptide assembly process is greatly influenced by statin drug use. The inevitability of dolichol inhibition, secondary to reductase blocking of the mevalonate pathway by statins, has been known to drug company biochemists from the very beginning of this multi-billion-dollar industry, but ignored almost completely by everyone else.

Even physicians get a smattering of this in medical school biochemistry, but all memory is usually lost by the time of graduation. Drug company management must have known of this problem to come for dolichol's role in our glycolysis and glycoprotein formation has been studied for many years and is well known to researchers in the field.

During the assembly of the peptide strand within the ER, sugars are added, thereby converting the product into glycoproteins. The usual sugars found in glycoproteins are glucose, galactose, mannose, fucose, N-acetyl galactosamine, N-acetyl glucosamine and N-acetyl neuraminic acid. The most frequently found sugar in this process is mannose. Their purpose is to broaden the versatility of the evolving protein structure by designating points and direction of protein folding — in this field of study, structure is function.

The final role depends on the protein structure. Just using proteins can give hundreds of options, but the addition of these sugars to the protein strand gives tens of thousands of structural options. It is this almost unlimited range of structural options that gives humans our tremendous range of behavioural and emotional reactions. This process, too, is orchestrated by dolichol in its preparation of the final protein structure.

This dolichol-mediated process is involved in neuropeptide formation and cell communication, cell identification and immune system functions. This complex role is such that almost anything can be expected when dolichols are deficient. Altered emotional and behavioral reactions associated with statin use are likely explained by altered neuropeptide formation.

The reality of dolichol inhibition by statins is thoroughly documented. The role of dolichols in the process of glycoprotein synthesis is also thoroughly documented. [1]

The pharmaceutical industry threw caution to the wind years ago when the national priority to lower cholesterol so fogged their minds that they (the medical, pharmaceutical and food industry) focused just on the cholesterol branch of the mevalonate pathway and completely disregarded the important consequences of collateral damage to the other main branches of our tree from statin drugs. The predictable result of all this has been a bizarre spectrum of statin associated side effects ranging from cognitive, to myotoxic, neurotoxic, neurodegenerative and behavioral.

I have been talking of the consequences of statin associated dolichol inhibition for years now, calling attention to the importance of this substance in neuropeptide formation and our feelings of thought, sensation and emotion. I have pointed at dolichol inhibition as a possible cause of statin associated behavioral side effects, such as irritability, hostility and depression.

Now, however, I have learned that this assembly of peptide fragments within the endoplasmic reticulum of every cell in our bodies is only a small part of dolichol's contribution. For it is here, in the heart of every cell, that our saccharides (sugars) are attached to proteins and lipids to give a far broader range of diversity and information transfer than either protein or lipid alone. This process is called glycolysis.

No longer do we consider these sugars as just simple fuel. The effects of these vital sugars on the resulting peptide structure being created in the endoplasmic reticulum and companion piece, the Golgi apparatus, is just short of miraculous. This attachment of sugars, this glycolysis, is completely dependent on dolichol's orchestration.

Throw in a statin and what do you have? An inevitable inhibition of dolichol (at times, probably roughly comparable to the degree of cholesterol inhibition). The resulting effect upon the body of this dolichol theft is completely unpredictable, for this is the very center of cell communication and immunodefense. Statin damage is often additive to pre-existing impairment of glycolysis from aging, disease and poor nutrition.

Dolichols may well be just as important as CoQ10 in this unfortunate game of statin roulette that Big Pharma has placed us in. Unfortunately, dolichol is not widely available as a supplement although several products are in development.

The effects of dolichols take place in the tiny micro-factories within each of our cells known as the endoplasmic reticulum (ER) and Golgi apparatus.[1] These are almost magical structures, responsible for progressive assembly of amino acid building blocks into long chains known as peptides.

This is the place of glycobiology. This is where our vital sugars are attached to give a truly extraordinary enhancement of cell communication and peptide effect. Without adequate dolichol bioavailability, neuropeptide formation, cell messaging and immunodefense are all potentially compromised.

There is no handy physiological number to measure dolichol deficiency as we have for cholesterol or CoQ10 levels. One must judge dolichol effect clinically on the basis of signs and symptoms.

The great variation of biologic properties that sugars offer to proteins as the peptide strands are being assembled is the strength of diversity, with virtually unlimited combinations of attachments thereby possible.

Molecular biologists have calculated that four amino acids alone can produce 24 different structural combinations of the resulting peptide strand. The addition of just four biologically active sugars, with their multiple points of attachments, can result in 124,000 possible structural combinations of the resulting glycoprotein strand.

This incredible specificity of design is a major strength of sugars with each variation of structure allowing a functional change. Think of the varying capacities for rage, love and envy of our neurohormones, all dependent on subtle variations of molecular structure.

For the purpose of mitochondrial maintenance, dolichols are absolutely vital to correct the daily load of oxidative damage our DNA must face, especially our mitochondrial DNA (it has a close proximity to oxygen for energy needs). Our daily assault by energetic radicals is a surprise to most.

We are living on the edge of extreme dependency upon both CoQ10 and dolichols. Our bioavailability of CoQ10 helps to minimize the oxidative damage because of its antioxidant effect, and the job of dolichols is to correct the damage missed by our CoQ10 defense. The glycohydrolases are vital to identify and correct each of the many thousands of DNA hits that occur daily.[2]

Imagine, even on a normal day we have tens of thousands of these errors to prevent and/or correct. It makes one cringe a bit just to think of using a statin drug, having the effect of inhibiting both CoQ10 and dolichols by its inevitable mevalonate blockade — a deadly double whammy, directly impacting our natural antioxidant defenses.

Another major area of glycoprotein function is in cellular identification and cell signaling, where sugar molecules on the cell's surface have the critical role of determining self from non-self, damaged versus healthy cells or inflamed tissue, which needs to be addressed.

Our immune system is strongly dependent upon this role of sugars. The structure of these surface molecules is characteristic of that cell and that cell only, giving each cell a virtual identification tag. Not only is this the basis of our immuno-defense reaction, it is vitally necessary even in such a basic function as blood grouping.

The key to blood transfusion is the ABO compatibility match between donor and receiver. The only difference between type O and types A and B is that the surface glycoproteins of type A and B contain one extra sugar molecule. Furthermore, the only difference between types A and B is in the sugar at one end of the molecular complex. Type A has an extra acetyl group, lacking on type B. All are determined by glycoproteins.

Finally, our glycoproteins are gatekeepers to the cells, regulating the transfer of ions of sodium, potassium, chloride and calcium through the cell membrane. Only recently has cystic fibrosis been identified as dependent upon a glycoprotein regulator responsible for the viscosity of the mucus within the tiny respiratory airways and pancreatic tubules.

Neutrophils, macrophages and natural killer cells are the foot soldiers; our first line of defense against injury and infection. They use glycoprotein matching to identify problem cells. They attack only those cells not having proper identification.

B-lymphocytes produce our antibodies and our T-lymphocytes engulf and destroy invaders, much like our foot soldiers just mentioned, but in a much more organized manner, seeking to destroy anything alien. This function is again dependent upon the basis of proper glycoprotein identification. Even our cytokines, such as interleukin, tumor necrosis factor and interferons, are dependent upon glycoproteins for activation.

Ordinarily, a normal healthy body produces its own supply of these biologically active sugars. Glucose and galactose are readily available in most diets and our bodies readily convert them into the other necessary sugars, but this conversion process is complex, energy dependent and prone to error.

Clearly, this description of the glycoprotein process, available in any standard biochemistry reference, suggests a primary role for mannose in this process, but mannose never works alone. All members of the biologically active family of sugars must be available and sufficient in an amount for the task at hand.

Mention has already been made of the inevitability of dolichol inhibition by the use of statin drugs. This process, like CoQ10 synthesis, is not something that may happen when statins inhibit our cellular mevalonate pathway — it is inevitable.

There is no disputing the ability of statin drugs to inhibit dolichol synthesis. Therefore, impacts on the mechanisms of glycoprotein action described above are inevitable.

Dolichol supervised attachments of sugars to the growing peptide chain is of major concern, for this is the stuff of neuropeptide formation. The types of protein and their sequence and folding characteristics are what determine the function of that particular peptide link.

One combination gives love, another hate, with hundreds of subtle values in between. Once formation of a peptide message strand is complete, the Golgi apparatus packages the product in a vesicle for safe keeping while traveling down the axon of a nerve to a synapse where they are stored until released.

The ultimate effect of this magic cluster of chemicals owes much to specific sugars and their points of attachment. The makeup of the proteins is of vast importance but it is the sugars which give it the rich spectrum of associated feelings, the subtle tones of guilt and fear that can accompany either love or hate.

We human creatures soon come to understand our emotional complexity, our subtle interplay of grays on more gray. Rarely are things black or white. This is the music of our glycoprotein instruments, playing to their dolichol director. The contribution of just this neuropeptide role boggles the mind in its complexity and challenge to measure. Just think of it; every thought, sensation or emotion the product of a specific neuropeptide linkage.[3]

Fully 20% of the total adverse reports for statin drugs include such symptoms as aggressiveness, hostility, sensitivity, paranoia, depression, sleep disturbances, suicidal ideation, suicides, homicidal ideation and "road rage" type behavior.

Men and women will state, "That is not the person I married." They mean this in the context of a fundamental and very real change in underlying personality, not some transient response based on a moment of anger. Physicians have even filed assault charges on patients who have no memory of the assault, remembering only that the doctor had been paying no attention to their complaints of memory loss and muscle pain.

The effects on cell messaging and immuno-responsiveness are just as complex if not more so. At this point in our understanding, it is impossible to predict the full spectrum of body systems potentially influenced by dolichols.

References for:
Dolichols, Statins and Personality Change

1. http://themedicalbiochemistrypage.org/glycoproteins.php

2. http://en.wikipedia.org/wiki/DNA_repair

3. Candace B. Pert - Molecules of emotion, Scribner, New York, 1997

Dolichols, Statins and Personality Change
Chapter Summary and Key Points.

- Proteins are synthesized within the membranes of the endoplasmic reticulum within each of our cells.

- Amino acids are linked together into a peptide with each peptide responsible for a diverse range of functions.

- This entire process is orchestrated by dolichols in the form of dolichol phosphate.

- The peptide assembly process is greatly influenced by statin drug use due to the inevitability of dolichol inhibition, secondary to reductase blocking of the mevalonate pathway by statins.

- It is the almost unlimited range of protein structural options that gives humans their tremendous range of behavioral and emotional reactions.

- Altered emotional and behavioral reactions associated with statin use are likely explained by altered neuropeptide formation.

- The national priority to lower cholesterol so fogged the minds of the medical, pharmaceutical and food industries that they completely disregarded the important consequences of collateral damage from statin drugs.

- In the heart of every cell, saccharides (sugars) are attached to proteins and lipids to give a far broader range of diversity and information transfer than either protein or lipid alone in a process called glycolysis.

- This attachment of sugars, this glycolysis, is completely dependent on dolichol's orchestration.

- Adding a statin provides an inevitable inhibition of dolichol.

- Statin damage is often additive to pre-existing impairment of glycolysis from aging, disease and poor nutrition.

- Dolichols may well be fully as important as CoQ10.

- The effects of dolichols take place in the endoplasmic reticulum and Golgi apparatus.

- There is no number to measure dolichol deficiency as we have for cholesterol or CoQ10 levels.

- One must judge dolichol effect clinically on the basis of signs and symptoms.

- For the purpose of mitochondrial maintenance, dolichols are absolutely vital to correct the daily load of oxidative damage our DNA must face.

- CoQ10 helps to minimize oxidative damage because of its antioxidant effect and dolichols correct the damage missed by our CoQ10 defense.

- On a normal day, we have tens of thousands of DNA errors to prevent and/or correct.

- Statin drugs, having the effect of inhibiting both CoQ10 and dolichols, directly impact our natural antioxidant defenses.

- The only difference between blood type O and types A and B is that the surface glycoproteins of type A and B contain one extra sugar molecule.

- The only difference between blood types A and B is in the sugar at one end of the molecular complex.

- All blood types are determined by glycoproteins.

- Neutrophils, macrophages and natural killer cells are the first line of defense against injury and infection. They use glycoprotein matching to identify problem cells.

- B-lymphocytes produce our antibodies and our T-lymphocytes engulf and destroy invaders, this function is dependent upon proper glycoprotein identification.

- There is no disputing the ability of statin drugs to inhibit dolichol synthesis, therefore impacts on the mechanisms of glycoprotein action are inevitable.

- Dolichol supervised attachments of sugars to the growing peptide chain is of major concern for one combination gives love, another hate, with hundreds of subtle values in between.

- Fully 20% of the total adverse reports for statin drugs include such symptoms as aggressiveness, hostility, sensitivity, paranoia, depression, sleep disturbances, suicidal ideation, suicides, homicidal ideation and "road rage" type behavior.

From CoQ10 Inhibition to Mitochondrial Mutations

I have written in the past of the association of statin drug use with such alarming adverse responses as transient global amnesia, behavioral and emotional change, peripheral neuropathies, myopathies and a neuromuscular degenerative condition resembling ALS. As serious as these conditions are, there are equally significant newly recognized effects of statin use: mitochondrial mutations.

We now realize one of the most serious side effects of statin drugs is their tendency to increase mitochondrial mutations, thereby contributing to premature aging and the onset of chronic conditions commonly associated with the aging process. This disastrous adverse response is the predictable consequence of CoQ10 and dolichol inhibition.

As I wrote earlier in this book, the reductase step of the mevalonate pathway that statins inhibit inevitably inhibits vital substances such as CoQ10, dolichols and selenoproteins and even normal phosphorylation. The process is inescapable.

Most of us have no awareness of just how critical CoQ10 is to our function; after the age of 50 we become increasingly unable to synthesize it and must depend almost entirely on what we take in by mouth. Dietary CoQ10 for most people is usually inadequate as the richest food sources are not widely consumed — beef and chicken hearts and livers. Therefore, supplements become an increasingly important source of CoQ10 as we age.

Even on our good days, mitochondrial mutations occur by the tens of thousands. They are an inevitable consequence of normal metabolic activity. The "reactive oxygen species" (ROS) — such as peroxidases and hydroxyl radicals — are produced as a byproduct of metabolism and desperately seek electrons to balance their electrical state. It is this "stealing" of electrons from adjacent tissue, including DNA strands, that causes the damage. We have evolved a very efficient anti-oxidative system for the purpose of minimizing this electron theft. Included in this system are such enzymes as superoxide dismutase and glutathione, and such non-enzymatic substances as coenzyme Q10 and vitamins C and E.

Although CoQ10 has plenty of help in its antioxidant role, I stress CoQ10's special importance because of its location within the mitochondria as a vital component of both complex one and complex two of the mitochondria's electron transfer sequence. What better location for the job at hand than being physically there, where the action is occurring.

CoQ10 not only is a vital component in this process of energy formation, it is also superbly placed for its powerful antioxidant function. In concert with the other members of this protective system, CoQ10 suffices to keep oxidative damage to a minimum. The DNA lesions that finally occur after the neutralizing effects of our legions of antioxidant warriors are then identified and corrected by another protective system of amazing efficiency.

Tens of thousands of DNA lesions occur daily despite all our antioxidant system can do, and is a sobering reality of the body seeking the best solution for meeting environmental change. Fortunately, most of these errors never make it beyond the next cell division, at which point they are replaced naturally by normal configurations. But the gradual buildup of these DNA errors can result in progressive loss of functional DNA, a frequent cause of chronic disease and the usual cause of aging.

Most of the serious damage is to our bases, those four amino acids: adenine, cytosine, thymine and guanine, comprising our DNA strands. Some of the oxidative damage can be reversed simply by direct chemical means. Far more important to us is the base excision repair process, in which faulty bases must be excised and replaced by correct ones.

This is one of the major repair requirements, occurring tens of thousands of times daily, and each one requiring a specific glycohydrolase. Since glycohydrolase is one of our ubiquitous glycoproteins, requiring dolichols for synthesis, one must consider the possibility of altered glycohydrolase availability with statin use. Please understand that the effect I am writing about is not some rare, remotely possible event. Mevalonate blockade of varying degrees is inevitable when statins are used.

The only escape from the consequences of this inhibition is the presence of pathway alternatives to the usual mevalonate one for synthesis of CoQ10, dolichols or even cholesterol. Obviously, many individuals take statins with apparent impunity and serum cholesterol sometimes does not respond to a statin at all. Both scenarios suggest the presence of alternative pathways for synthesis. If this is true for cholesterol, it is true for all other biochemicals equally dependent upon the mevalonate pathway. In my 23 years of clinical medicine I soon discovered that I was fortunate if five out of every ten patients exhibited the expected response to a given medicine. The possible presence of yet to be discovered alternative pathways reflects what doctors have always known: even though we look alike and act alike, we are all different in terms of underlying biochemistry.

Other than for these considerations, mevalonate blockade has to occur with statin use and is the cause of the overwhelming majority of adverse reactions. The consequence of CoQ10 and dolichol inhibition is mitochondrial damage. It is inescapable, and every doctor using or recommending these drugs must understand this.

Tens of thousands of statin users have been damaged by statins. I suspect that mitochondrial damage is the principle cause of most of the conditions involved. CoQ10 alone is rarely successful in treating these conditions, although it appears to be a primary factor in causation. Treatment efforts should include doing what seems reasonable to help reverse this process.

At this point no one can say this approach will definitely reverse the process, or even help, but we must keep in mind that conventional medicine has little to offer. No one can say this will not work until the concept has been thoroughly tested. The reason that no trials have been done as yet is largely because statin causation has been generally dismissed by doctors. The concept of inevitable mitochondrial damage from the use of reductase inhibitors is alien to most clinicians because they have not felt the need to review the biochemistry. A reasonable goal appears to be the restoration of mitochondrial function by whatever means are available.

For those statin victims desiring background information on their statin-associated myopathy, neuropathy, ALS-like condition, and even cognitive dysfunction, what I present here should suffice, for this condition can occur in any tissue: muscle, nerve, or brain. The diminished bioavailability of intracellular CoQ10 and dolichols associated with the use of statins has the potential for seriously increasing oxidative damage and DNA mutations.

The logical consequence of this is premature aging and the progressive development of such chronic conditions of aging as muscle weakness, burning pain and incoordination and faulty memory; exactly what we are seeing in tens of thousands of statin users. The clinical responses we are seeing from this process of progressive mitochondrial damage are highly variable, more of a spectrum than any predictable, precise display of symptoms.

We first have to accept that most statin users appear to do quite well on statins. This tells me that in some people the mevalonate pathway must take several different forms or by-pass channels, if you will, that allow sufficient CoQ10, dolichols, selenoproteins, and so forth to be available, despite blockade of the basic mevalonate pathway.

We also find that some persons are completely unresponsive to statins, strongly supporting this possible presence of alternative pathways. We can also say that premature aging and the earliest forms of neuropathy and myopathy may not yet be clinically apparent. Dull aches, slight numbness, senior moments and personality change can all be so minor as to escape recognition as possibly significant, so at least some of those who appear to be tolerant may actually have subclinical decrement and are unaware of a possible relationship with statin use.

Just as we have to accept the fact that many, even most patients appear tolerant to statins, thousands of other people have been disabled by statins.

I have generally categorized the symptoms as cognitive, emotional, neuropathic, myopathic and neurodegenerative, but in reality there is much overlap. And hovering above all of these categories is the frequent presentation of tiredness and easy fatigability, pointing directly at deficient energy. Fatigue is the end result of a lack of adenosine triphosphate (ATP), so with sufficient mitochondrial damage, fatigue becomes inevitable.

The cognitive manifestations of statins may be just episodes of transient global amnesia, or increasing confusion, disorientation and forgetfulness or progressive dementia, which could be called Alzheimer's-like, differing only in underlying pathology. Only when one stops the statins and sees regression of symptoms can the true cause be inferred.

So an individual can present with any one or all of these symptoms. It all depends upon what kind of cell body tissue is the more involved with mitochondrial deterioration. Every cell comes equipped with mitochondria, the energy producers of the cell. The cells of slowly metabolizing tissue may be composed of only a few mitochondria because its energy needs are minimal. Muscle, heart and brain cells come equipped with hundreds of mitochondria because of the urgency of their metabolic demand.

From CoQ10 Inhibition to Mitochondrial Mutations
Chapter Summary and Key Points.

- One of the most serious side effects of statin drugs is their tendency to increase mitochondrial mutations, thereby contributing to premature aging.

- This disastrous adverse response is the predictable consequence of CoQ10 and dolichol inhibition.

- After the age of 50 we become increasingly unable to synthesize CoQ10.

- CoQ10 is found only in very small amounts in the average diet.

- Tens of thousands of mitochondrial mutations occur every day.

- CoQ10 is a component of the body's antioxidant system.

- Thousands of DNA lesions occur daily despite our antioxidant system.

- The gradual buildup of these DNA errors can result in progressive loss of functional DNA.

- Mevalonate blockade of varying degrees is inevitable when statins are used.

- The consequence of CoQ10 and dolichol inhibition is mitochondrial damage plus increased oxidative damage and DNA mutations.

- With sufficient mitochondrial damage, fatigue becomes inevitable.

- Every cell comes equipped with mitochondria, the energy producers of the cell.

- Muscle, heart and brain cells have hundreds of mitochondria because of their metabolic demand.

Mitochondrial Mutations: Could Mevalonate Help?

Nearly three decades after the first statin was marketed, statin researchers are just beginning to define the mechanisms whereby statin drugs can cause serious side effects. I have been reporting side effects for at least fifteen years now, but in this era of "statins can do no wrong," only a few have listened.

The drug companies had us so distracted with misinformation and data manipulation that side-effect truths were kept hidden. Now research scientists are reporting in their journals what some have been predicting for years.

Do-Sim Park and others, of South Korea's University School of Medicine, published in the peer-reviewed medical journal *Acta Oto-Laryngologic*[1], their observations that the commonly used statin drug, Zocor® (simvastatin), induces death of cochlear neurons (nerves in the ear that carry sounds to the brain).

In this technically very neat and straight-forward piece of research, cell cultures consisting of neurons from the organs of hearing of experimental animals were treated with Zocor in the absence or presence of mevalonate. Subsequent exposure to Zocor caused extensive degenerative changes in this neurologic tissue, including neuronal cell death. All of these effects were abolished by mevalonate treatment.

As with all other statins, Zocor is a HMG-CoA reductase inhibitor, the effect of which has been to block the mevalonate pathway, contributing to cell damage and death. Giving mevalonate prevented these changes, showing they were caused by mevalonate blockade. This is what I mean by neat and technically straight-forward.

For many years now, I have been saying that statins cause mevalonate blockade and have postulated this mechanism of action for many of the side effects of statin drug use. Dr. Park and his team have shown this to be correct.

But Dr. Park's research is not the only one to demonstrate the reversibility of statin damage with mevalonate. Hundreds of studies have reported this effect of mevalonate on statins. It is now an accepted indicator of statin causation — the ability of mevalonate to reverse the change.

The astute observer will immediately pick up on this reversibility factor of mevalonate for its possible benefit in statin damage. The only evidence in support of this possibility is the hundreds of reports of mevalonate use to reverse statin induced blockade. If a statin induces a change via mevalonate inhibition, then mevalonate given at some reasonable time period afterwards may reverse it, showing statin causality and suggesting a possible statin damage treatment option.

The time period between administering the statin and administering the mevalonate is likely a critical one and in the studies available to me, the mevalonate has been given immediately afterwards. For cognitive damage, where the causative factor is inhibition of cholesterol synthesis leading to amnesia, confusion, disorientation and extreme forgetfulness, I suspect the effect of mevalonate supplementation would be an almost immediate restoration of glial cell cholesterol synthesis.

However, the type of damage done by the reduction of such substances as CoQ10 and dolichols is something else entirely. CoQ10 has a vital antioxidant role for our mitochondria. Because of the intimate inclusion of CoQ10 in complexes I and II, the result of abrupt inhibition of CoQ10 bioavailability through mevalonate blockade leads to abrupt loss of antioxidant effectiveness. This allows excess numbers of energetic radicals to access adjacent DNA, causing the rapid accumulation of damaged mitochondrial DNA.

The resulting clinical evidence might ultimately be neuropathy or myopathy depending on the type of tissue primarily affected. Supplementing with mevalonate at this point might be like the proverbial locking the barn door after the horse has bolted — the damage has already been done. But it is premature to make any kind of prediction concerning mevalonate effectiveness in treatment of these kinds of conditions because we do not yet have the data. These data are badly needed.

Concerning the inhibition of dolichol associated with statin use for many people, the role of dolichol in formulating glycoprotein neurohormones must be considered. The likely clinical consequences of this are the many cases of emotional and behavioral adverse reactions that have been reported associated with the use of statins.

Dr. Golomb of the University of California, San Diego (UCSD) School of Medicine as part of a U.S. National Institutes of Health (NIH) funded statin study, has reported on the hostility/aggression/road rage syndrome associated with statin use.[2]

The full spectrum of symptoms reported range from aggressiveness and irritability to paranoia and depression, to homicidal and suicidal ideation, to actual homicides and suicides. What would be the effect of mevalonate supplementation on someone with these kinds of symptoms? I would hope for a prompt return to normal neurohormone synthesis but, of course, we must have the data to support this idea.

References for:
Mitochondrial Mutations: Could Mevalonate Help?

1. Park, Do-Sim. Reversal of statin induced ganglion with mevalonate in murine model. A*cta Oto-laryngologica* 129 (2);155-167, 2009

2. Golomb, B. and others. Severe irritability associated with statin cholesterol-lowering drugs. *QJM* 97, 229-235, 2004.

Mitochondrial Mutations: Could Mevalonate Help?
Chapter Summary and Key Points.

- Statins cause mevalonate blockade and this appears to be the source of many of the side effects of statins.

- Blockade of mevalonate from statins has been reversed by adding mevalonate in studies.

- Mevalonate given at some reasonable time period after adding a statin may offer a possible statin damage treatment option.

- In studies I have reviewed, mevalonate was given immediately after the statin was administered.

- The type of damage done by the reduction of such substances as CoQ10 and dolichols is something else entirely and independent of mevalonate.

- It is premature to make any kind of prediction concerning mevalonate effectiveness in treatment of statin damage because we do not yet have the data.

Anti-Oxidation and Mitochondrial Damage

"You can't live with it and you can't live without it." This statement comes very close to describing our love/hate relationship with the oxygen in the air around us. On one hand, oxygen is absolutely vital for life as the basis for energy production. On the other hand, the oxidizing tendency of oxygen with its production of highly energetic radicals, has necessitated the evolution of our powerful antioxidant system to minimize the oxidative damage suffered by our tissues and, more importantly, our mitochondrial DNA.

Our nuclear DNA is quite well protected compared with that of our mitochondria. Wrapped in a histone barrier, with a far more aggressive anti-inflammatory capacity, and outside the daily skirmish with oxygen, nuclear DNA is mostly protected from oxidative harm.

Most textbooks define oxidation as a chemical reaction that often produces damaging free radicals by the transfer of electrons. Antioxidants help remove these free radicals, thereby minimizing tissue damage.[1] Some examples of antioxidants are glutathione, vitamins C and A, coenzyme Q10, superoxide dismutase, catalase and various peroxidases. Any substance that inhibits the bioavailability of antioxidants, such as the inhibitory effect of statin drugs on coenzyme Q10, may damage our DNA. Especially vulnerable, because of its immediate proximity to high oxygen levels, is our mitochondrial DNA.

The initial interest in oxidation began because of the need to prevent the damage from rust. Soon this interest was extended to studying the process of preventing rancidity of fats in storage. But it was the antioxidant activity of vitamins A, C and E that revolutionized the field and pointed to the critical role of antioxidants in human biochemistry.

The use of oxygen, as part of the process for generating metabolic energy, produces highly energetic radicals known as "reactive oxygen species" (ROS). Since reactive oxygen species do have some useful functions in cells, the function of antioxidant systems is not to remove oxidants entirely, but instead to keep them at an optimum level. The reactive oxygen species produced in cells include hydrogen peroxide, hypochlorous acid, and free radicals such as the hydroxyl radical and the superoxide ion. These oxidants can damage cells by starting chemical chain reactions such as lipid peroxidation, or by oxidizing DNA or proteins. Damage to DNA can cause mutations, if this damage is not reversed by DNA repair mechanisms.

Of particular importance in this process is the reduction of ubiquinol (coenzyme Q10) in complex III, where electrons can jump directly to oxygen, forming superoxide ions instead of taking the usual electron transfer path. These interactions that form oxidants are complex and many are still not completely understood.

Antioxidants have both independent and interdependent effects. While their individual, independent actions are quite well established, the interdependent actions, in many cases, remain to be explained. The action of one antioxidant may depend upon the availability and proper concentration of another antioxidant, as well as its own special sensitivity to a particular reactive oxygen species and its own concentration. Other antioxidants will depend upon the bioavailability of such elements as selenium to have proper activity. Selenium has long been known to function as an antioxidant nutrient, despite completely lacking in such activity by itself.

Although the antioxidants as a group are similar in their reducing effects, many have individual characteristics that are important to note in dealing with reactive oxygen species. Ascorbic acid (one form of vitamin C) functions as a reducing agent and is only available naturally from dietary sources.

Our inability to synthesize this substance is of critical importance when the elderly or infirm are unable to get sufficient amounts from dietary sources alone. Supplementation is vital in many cases and the amounts are frequently inadequate. The need for this vitamin can change rapidly under stress conditions. It functions only as a reducing agent with effects on reactive oxygen species that, despite numerous studies, remain theoretical.

Another important antioxidant, glutathione, shares vitamin C's role of functioning as a reducing agent. Glutathione is not required in the diet and is instead readily synthesized in our cells. Due to its usual high tissue concentration, glutathione is one of the most important cellular antioxidants.

Most important of the glutathiones are the glutathione peroxidases, which contain four selenium co-factors, having a major role in hydrogen peroxide breakdown. Statins inhibit selenoprotein synthesis; glutathione reductase is a selenoprotein. This selenoprotein is responsible for maintaining the antioxidant glutathione in its reduced state to increase its antioxidant functions.

Melatonin, once reduced, cannot be recycled. After it has been oxidized, melatonin cannot revert to its former state because it forms several stable end products upon reacting with free radicals.

Melatonin is a powerful antioxidant that ordinarily is reliably synthesized in sufficient amounts by the body. It was only as recently as 1993 that the importance of melatonin as a powerful antioxidant was established. In addition, it has a long established role in the functioning of our biological clocks of day/night cycling. Melatonin crosses the blood-brain barrier giving it free access to our brains.

Melatonin is also a direct scavenger of nitric oxide, the hydroxyl radical, and the oxygen ion. The first metabolite of melatonin in the melatonin antioxidant pathway appears to be AFMK (acetyl-N-formyl-5-methoxykynurenamine), which has unusually effective antioxidant capacity, leading to a biochemical process known as the free radical scavenging cascade. This capacity is limited only to melatonin, distinguishing it as an unusually capable antioxidant.

Vitamin E has a few peculiarities that should be mentioned here. For most of the past 80 years, when anyone ordered or consumed vitamin E, they were using the tocopherol form. In the past fifteen years, the other form of vitamin E, the tocotrienol form with antioxidation effectiveness some 50 times greater than tocopherol, has been identified and developed.

The Annatto source, a South American plant, yields almost pure tocotrienol,[2] and in addition to its antioxidation role, appears to have the interesting metabolic actions of maintaining rather than blocking the mevalonate pathway. Like tocopherol, its action is primarily that of inhibiting lipid peroxidation (the oxidative degradation of lipids) but the full scope of activity regarding reactive oxygen species neutralization remains to be determined.

The enzyme superoxide dismutase (SOD) converts the oxidant, superoxide, into hydrogen peroxide, which is further converted to water. The enzyme catalase (that catalyzes hydrogen peroxide to its constituent parts of hydrogen and oxygen) and the peroxidases (a large family of enzymes also involved in catalyzing) all have complex interactions difficult to separate. Our cells are well supplied with SOD enzymes, most of which are combined with metallic co-factors. Manganese SOD is the combination most often present in our mitochondria.

The observation that our body is heavily supplied with a complex system of potentially interacting antioxidants documents the adverse effect of oxidation in our body. Yet numerous studies have been conducted by supplementing with one antioxidant or another with them failing to show a consistent effect.

For every study done documenting a positive contribution, another will appear in the literature refuting the results. Obviously antioxidants are critical to health and even life, yet we seem unable at this point to prove it. We need to know much more about the various actions and interactions of the antioxidants.

The importance of our inbuilt antioxidant system in serving to minimize the production of reactive oxygen species is well established. But because a substance is an antioxidant, even a powerful antioxidant such as vitamin C or tocotrienol, does not necessarily mean that particular substance is vital to the body's antioxidant function.

Those antioxidants that are vital are the ones that biochemists have thoroughly documented to be intimately involved in underlying biochemistry. No one can challenge the effectiveness of superoxide dismutases or glutathione and the necessity of their metallic co-factors.

Our mitochondria are well supplied with SOD enzymes and their manganese cofactor. Glutathiones, in the form of glutathione peroxidases with their selenium co-factors, have a major role in hydrogen peroxide breakdown. Additionally, melatonin appears to be very important, especially with its unique ability to trigger a "free radical scavenging cascade," and can anyone dispute CoQ10's critical role, especially with its placement in our mitochondria's complex one and two?

But what of vitamin C and vitamin E? In the hundreds of studies where supplemental use has failed to show significant effect, should we ask the question does the antioxidant chemical effect of a substance such as these vitamins automatically establish them as legitimate members of an antioxidant team? The question must be asked. I do not yet have the answer. However, I am completely convinced of the vital roles of superoxide dismutase, glutathione peroxidases, CoQ10 and melatonin.

Because of its high metabolic rate, the brain is particularly vulnerable to oxidative injury. This has triggered the evaluation of a number of different techniques for brain injury treatment in the form of analogues of both superoxide dismutase and glutathione, with some very promising early results supporting the concept that not all antioxidants may be equal.

There is no way to predict how any one person will respond to this progressive mitochondrial deterioration triggered by statins. It all depends on a roll of the dice. Therefore, a cognitively impaired victim may also present with emotional symptoms, painful neuropathy, disabling myopathy or an ALS-like manifestation.

References for:
Anti-Oxidation and Mitochondrial Damage

1. http://en.wikipedia.org/wiki/Reactive_oxygen_species

2. Tan, B and Mueller, A. Tocotrienols : Vitamin E beyond tocopherol. Watson R. AOCS Press, 2008

Anti-Oxidation and
Mitochondrial Damage
Chapter Summary and Key Points.

- Our antioxidant system minimizes the oxidative damage to mitochondrial DNA.

- Oxidation is a chemical reaction that often produces damaging free radicals.

- Antioxidants help remove free radicals.

- The inhibitory effect of statin drugs on coenzyme Q10 may damage DNA.

- The function of antioxidant systems is to keep oxidants at an optimum level.

- Damage to DNA can cause mutations.

- Antioxidants have both independent and interdependent effects.

- Just because a substance is an antioxidant, it does not necessarily mean that it is vital to the body's antioxidant function.

- Because of its high metabolic rate, the brain is particularly vulnerable to oxidative injury.

- There is no way to predict how any individual will respond to progressive mitochondrial deterioration triggered by statins.

Aging and Mitochondrial Mutations

In the past, I have cautioned about the use of statins for those with diabetes because of the report by Gaist of a much greater tendency for peripheral neuropathy in those taking statin drugs.[1] Since neuropathy is already a serious problem for diabetics, the effect of adding statins to their treatment program has always concerned me. Mitochondrial damage, the special focus here, raises the risk level of peripheral neuropathy for many people to excessive heights.

Previously, my work on researching statin drug side effects had led me only to the formidable blockade of the mevalonate pathway, with all that it entails. But to find that statins work their damage by still another mechanism is to add a whole new dimension to the word "serious". I can think of no greater pharmaceutical concern than a drug that interferes with our DNA, nuclear or mitochondrial. The barest hint of this mechanism of action of a drug should be sufficient to propel society's defenses to emergency alert.

Imagine a class of drugs with effects so subtle, that a decade may pass before society awakens to the truth? Do you remember thalidomide? Now, instead of birth defects, we have cognitive defects including increased senility, permanent peripheral neuropathy, chronic disabling neuro-muscular degeneration, and increased numbers of statin patients with neuro-degenerative diseases such as Parkinsonism, Alzheimer's disease and ALS-like symptoms. All these are casually dismissed in doctor's offices as old age and coincidence. For the most part these are not coincidences, and dismissal without thorough investigation is unacceptable.

Abundant research evidence now exists in the medical literature indicating that diminished mitochondrial function, through excess oxidation, occurs inevitably as we age,[2] and is also a major factor in fatiguing illnesses common to the elderly — as well as the process of aging itself. This is a reflection of progressive loss of efficiency in the electron transport chain. This degradation appears to be naturally associated with the process of aging, and is the primary mechanism in the fatigue of many chronic diseases, especially those of ALS and the tauopathies[3] — those neurodegenerative conditions believed to be associated with excess tau protein production.

Included in this long list of specific disease syndromes are Parkinsonism, frontotemporal dementia and multiple system atrophy, all reported to me by people taking statins. The long, filamentous protein strands that characterize this collection of diseases likely reflects, at least in part, altered nuclear DNA damage, which can be expected to occur along with that of mitochondrial DNA.

One of the most important changes in tissues and cells that occur during aging and chronic degenerative disease, is accumulated oxidative damage due to cellular reactive oxygen species (ROS). ROS are oxidative, as well as free radical oxygen and nitrogen containing molecules, such as nitric oxide, and hydroxide radicals, and other molecules.

Critical targets of ROS are the genetic apparatus, with its susceptibility to mutations, and cellular membranes. In the latter case, oxidation can affect lipid fluidity, permeability and membrane function. Similar changes occur in fatiguing illnesses, such as chronic fatigue syndrome (CFS) and heart failure, where patients show increased susceptibility to oxidative stress by decreased adenosine triphosphate (ATP) synthesis.

The major consequence of excess oxidation is excess mitochondrial damage. Not only does the rate of damage increase as we age, but the ability of our bodies to identify and replace mitochondrial DNA defects degrades.

A major contributor to this excess accumulation of oxidative damage is coenzyme Q10 deficiency — the principal antioxidant to mitochondrial function. Our ability to synthesize CoQ10 progressively falls with age, and by midlife most of us are completely dependent on external sources of this vital substance. It is difficult to overstate the importance of this powerful antioxidant, for in addition to its role as a suppressor of ROS over-abundance, it is also vital for cell wall integrity, and is a necessary element of our electron transport system. "No CoQ10, no cellular energy," says it all.

Few seniors have the CoQ10 adequacy of their youth. Supplementation is not only important for this group, but critical for most. As we have learned elsewhere in this book, the use of statin drugs greatly increases this problem. To reduce cholesterol, statin drugs block the mevalonate pathway, critical to the synthesis of such vital substances as CoQ10 and dolichols.

Dolichols are critical to the synthesis of glycoproteins; their importance is difficult to overstate.[4] Made in the endoplasmic reticulum in almost every cell in our bodies, glycoproteins comprise the neuropeptide molecules of emotion, cell identification, and cell communication. Glycoproteins also play a vital role in the immune system.

The ability to synthesize dolichols progressively falls off with time in most people, due to genetic predisposition, nutritional factors, and prior disease. Many people in midlife are not all that different from statin users, in that dolichol insufficiency may be present. This is another reason why from mid-life on, strange things begin to happen in our bodies, all of them bad. This is another reason why statin users and seniors are all in the same boat regarding mitochondrial mutations.

With respect to mitochondrial mutations, a specific glycohydrolase, a member of the glycoprotein family, must be produced for each of the thousands of mitochondrial DNA errors that need to be corrected daily. This entire operation is orchestrated by dolichols. Any interference with the availability of dolichols must compromise this critical repairing function, adding to the damage and mutation load.

This past decade has seen major advances in defining the role of mitochondrial damage in aging and disease. The components of our energy equation are now well known. Ninety percent (34 of the 38 moles) of ATP, generated in a cell during oxidation of one mole of glucose, is highly dependent upon the availability of CoQ10, which is used to generate a "proton gradient" across the inner mitochondrial membrane. This gradient is what moves electrons "downhill," so that the enzyme ATP synthase literally "spins" to make ATP. This ATP-generating and CoQ10 dependent process is called "electron transport" or "oxidative-level phosphorylation."

As glucose is broken down via oxidation, hydrogen atoms are metabolized or "broken off" and "picked up" by vitamins B3 (niacin) and B2 (riboflavin), which are reduced, respectively, to form NADH and FADH2. (The hydrogen atoms "H" in NADH and H2 in FADH2 will, provided CoQ10 is present in the mitochondria, be converted into ATP). In medical school, we all memorized NADH and FADH2 as components of the Krebs cycle (part of oxidation) without realizing that these are reduced forms of niacin and riboflavin, common B vitamins.

The bottom line is this. Without the presence of CoQ10, a proton gradient cannot be formed. Without a proton gradient, the entire ATP-generation process via oxidative phosphorylation (also known as electron transport) comes to a screeching halt. Our very life, which relies on the proper function of our cells, or more specifically the mitochondria of our cells, is dependent on the movement of electrons, and protection from free radical oxidation.

The resulting ill effects seen in some statin users include the following: mitochondrial mutations leading to permanent myopathy, neuropathy and neurodegenerative diseases, lack of energy leading to chronic fatigue and congestive heart failure, and lack of cell wall integrity leading to myopathy, rhabdomyolysis, neuropathy and hepatitis.

Because of the high energy demands of heart cells, each cell has many thousands of mitochondria to generate the necessary energy/ATP for proper cardiac function. A blockade of CoQ10, therefore, causes the greatest threat of loss of life in terms of the effect on the myocardium (the thickest layer of the heart muscle). This is not to minimize the reality that such a blockade of CoQ10 has a negative effect on every cell-type throughout the body.

Damage to mitochondrial components, mainly by ROS oxidation, can impair their ability to produce high energy molecules such as ATP. This occurs naturally with aging and during chronic illnesses, where the production of ROS can cause oxidative stress and cellular damage. The result is oxidation of lipids, proteins, and both cellular and mitochondrial DNA.

The integrity of mitochondrial membranes is critical to cell function and energy metabolism. When mitochondrial membrane lipids are damaged by oxidation, they must be repaired or replaced in order to maintain the production of cellular energy, to alleviate fatigue. During aging, and in many diseases including fatiguing illnesses, ROS-mediated accumulation of oxidized mitochondrial lipids occurs. The failure to repair or replace these damaged molecules, at a rate that exceeds their damage, results in impaired mitochondrial function.

Mitochondrial membrane damage, and subsequent dysfunction by ROS, can also lead to an increased rate of mitochondrial DNA modifications (especially mutations and deletions). The mitochondrial theory of aging proposes that aging, and the development of age-related degenerative diseases, are primarily the result of accumulated oxidative damage to mitochondrial membranes and DNA, over time. Restoration of mitochondrial membrane integrity, fluidity, and other properties, are essential for the optimal functioning of the electron transport chain.

The ability to control membrane lipid peroxidation (rancid fat from oxidation) and DNA damage, will likely play an important role in slowing down the development of age-related degenerative diseases. Antioxidants are currently under study for maintaining mitochondrial function and preventing fatigue, and could be an important part of treatment strategies in the future for chronic fatigue syndrome, and other fatiguing illnesses.

References for:
Aging and Mitochondrial Mutations.

1. Gaist, D. and others. Statins and the risk of polyneuropathy. *Neurology* 58;1333-1337, 2002

2. http://www.pnas.org/content/102/52/18769.full

3. http://en.wikipedia.org/wiki/Tauopathy

4. http://en.wikipedia.org/wiki/DNA_repair (glycoprotein synthesis section)

Aging and Mitochondrial Mutations
Chapter Summary and Key Points.

- Our antioxidant system minimizes the oxidative damage to mitochondrial DNA.

- Coenzyme Q10 is the principal antioxidant to mitochondrial function.

- Dolichols are critical to the synthesis of glycoproteins.

- Thousands of mitochondrial DNA errors must be corrected daily and is orchestrated by dolichols.

- The mitochondrial theory of aging proposes that aging is primarily the result of accumulated oxidative damage over time to mitochondrial membranes and DNA.

Mitochondrial Damage in Aging

In 2002, G. Vladutiu and others, announced in *Annals of Internal Medicine* the results of detailed studies on four myopathy (muscular disease) patients, all of whom had normal muscle enzyme test results.[1] This was one of the first studies to link statin use with myopathy without muscle enzyme abnormality.

This condition was manifested by lipid deposition in the muscle fibers, unusual staining characteristics of these muscle fibers, and the condition known as "ragged red fibers". These features were labeled as "statin myopathy" due to an underlying metabolic abnormality.

Although some of these findings may rarely occur in myofibrils (parallel threads that run the length of muscles) because of aging, the pattern of increased lipid deposition was distinctly unusual. The metabolic abnormalities were believed to reflect mitochondrial mutations as a consequence of statin use. It had previously been described as a respiratory chain defect associated with coenzyme Q10 deficiency.

Ragged red fiber disease was first used to describe a set of mitochondrial myopathies in 1972, because muscle fibers with enough abnormal mitochondria were colored red when viewed under a microscope, after modified trichrome staining. Ragged red fibers are an important marker for mitochondrial disease.

During the past two decades, much has been learned about mitochondrial myopathies and their association, not only with ragged red myofibrils, but also with a great variety of neuro-degenerative syndromes. In 1995, Rifai, Z. and others, after studying the frequency of ragged red fibers in muscle biopsy specimens, reported in the journal *Neurology* that the number of ragged red fibers increases with normal aging, and may reflect an age-related decline in muscle mitochondrial oxidative metabolism.[2] What was known then as "inclusion body myositis" consistently revealed ragged red myofibrils, marking it as secondary to a defect in the respiratory chain, and therefore metabolic in origin, rather than inflammatory.

During this time period, muscle CoQ10 was found to be deficient in these metabolic myopathy cases. This is clearly associated with the known inhibitory effect of statins on mevalonate derived CoQ10. Although CoQ10 plays a primary role in the energy equation of the body, it is also a powerful antioxidant that along with glutathione, helps to prevent excess buildup of free radicals. In the event of lack of availability of sufficient CoQ10 and glutathione, rapid mitochondrial mutation can be expected. The normal mutation rate for mitochondrial DNA is some 4-8 times that of somatic (body and organ) cells, so the effect of a lack of CoQ10 can severely increase the rate of mutation.

In 2003, Carvalho and others reported eight cases of statin associated myopathy with histologic (tissue) changes very similar to these earlier metabolic myopathy cases, including muscle biopsy evidence of ragged red myofibrils.[3] Some had elevated creatine kinase (CK) enzymes; many did not. There followed a host of reports of unusual statin-associated myopathies related with a large variety of brain and other organ defects.

Then we learned of "Mitochondrial Encephalopathy, Lactic Acidosis, and Stroke-like Episodes" (MELAS) associated with statin use, and a bewildering alphabet soup of other statin associated "cerebromyopathies," all expressing mitochondrial mutations, causing respiratory chain dysfunction. I have seen several instances of probable statin associated MELAS, but most doctors find it impossible to accept statin causation.

Nicolson and Ellithorpe reported in their paper, "Lipid Replacement and Antioxidant Nutritional Therapy for Restoring Mitochondrial Function and Reducing Fatigue in Chronic Fatigue Syndrome and other Fatiguing Illnesses," extensive studies on lipid replacement therapy for the chronic fatigue of aging and chronic illnesses.[4] Associated with their therapy, substantial reversals of fatigue have been documented. Their lipid replacement therapy emphasizes such fats as phosphatidyl choline and phosphatidyl inositol, combined with both linoleic (omega-6) and linolenic (omega-3) acids and other antioxidants.

Huang and Manton published a brilliant review of the role of oxidative damage in mitochondria during aging.[5] They reported that macromolecules, damaged by the oxidative process, accumulate with age in every organism examined; thus, oxidative damage is implicated in many human age-related diseases. With age, mitochondrial function declines and mitochondrial DNA mutations increase. They found that the Alzheimer's disease affected brain shows higher levels of oxidative damage to both proteins and lipids.

Huang and Manton also discovered that energetic radicals are involved in many diseases of the elderly, including Alzheimer's disease (AD) and Parkinson's disease (PD), as well as conditions affecting vision, such as cataracts and macular degeneration. Neurodegenerative diseases have been linked to mutations in mitochondrial DNA (mtDNA) and nuclear DNA (nDNA).

Evidence of mitochondrial dysfunction also exists for other neurodegenerative diseases such as degenerating and non-degenerating tissues of amyotrophic lateral sclerosis (ALS), subjects with progressive supranuclear palsy, multisystem atrophy and Huntington's disease. Numerous studies support the notion that oxidative damage to mtDNA, and mitochondrial respiratory function, are important contributors to human aging.

A few years ago, a friend of mine died of multiple system atrophy (MSA). This former Navy Seal was in his late forties and in excellent health, until shortly after a statin was started for mild cholesterol elevation. The real diagnosis came late, having been preceded by first, multiple sclerosis, and then, Lou Gehrig's disease.

He had been on a statin for only a year when symptoms first began, giving me considerable concern at the speed with which his progressive mitochondrial damage developed. Of course, a statin etiology could never be proven, but I seriously doubt Mother Nature could have moved that fast. I shake my head helplessly as these statin associated neurodegenerative cases accumulate.

Brierly, E.J. and others, reported in the *Annals of Neurology*, their study of elderly muscle tissue for mitochondrial mutations.[6] "In muscle tissue from normal elderly subjects, we show that there are muscle fibers with very low activity of cytochrome c oxidase, suggestive of a mitochondrial DNA (mtDNA) defect. In these cytochrome c oxidase-deficient fibers, we have found very high levels of mutant mtDNA. In addition, different mtDNA mutations are present in different fibers, which explains why there is a low overall incidence of an individual mutation in tissues from elderly subjects. These studies show a direct age-related correlation between a biochemical and genetic defect in normal human tissues, and that mtDNA abnormalities are involved in the aging process in human muscle."

Wei and Lee reported their findings that mitochondria act like a biosensor of oxidative stress, and they enable cells to undergo changes in aging and age-related diseases.[7] "It has recently been demonstrated, that impairment in mitochondrial respiration and oxidative phosphorylation, elicits an increase in oxidative stress, and causes a host of mtDNA rearrangements and deletions." They reviewed work done in the past few years to support their view that oxidative stress (oxidative damage), is a result of concurrent accumulation of mtDNA mutations and defective antioxidant enzymes in human aging.

In Halliwell's review article, "Role of free radicals in the neurodegenerative diseases: therapeutic implications for antioxidant treatment," he reports that oxidative stress has been extensively studied in neurologic disease, including Alzheimer's disease, Parkinson's disease, multiple sclerosis, ALS, AIDS, dementia, and so on.[8]

This is not surprising since the brain is especially susceptible to oxidative stress, and subsequent damage to cells including cell death. In a disease such as Alzheimer's, oxidative stress and oxidative damage is felt to play a key role in the loss of neurons, and the progression to dementia.

Xu and Finkel, on explaining a role for mitochondria as potential regulators of cellular life span, reported that "growing evidence supports the concept that mitochondrial metabolism and reactive oxygen species (ROS) play a major role in aging and determination of an organism's life span."[9]

Lin and others reported on the high burden of mitochondrial DNA mutations in Alzheimer's.[10]

In a paper titled, "Oxidative stress causes heart failure with impaired mitochondrial respiration", H. Nojiri and others reported that elderly people, "insidiously manifest the symptoms of heart failure, such as dyspnea and/or physical disabilities in an age-dependent manner.[11] We here present a bona fide model for human cardiac failure with oxidative stress valuable for therapeutic interventions."

Keshav K. Singh, in a paper titled, "Mitochondria Damage Checkpoint, Aging, and Cancer," reports growing evidence supporting the progressive decline in mitochondrial function with age.[12] "Mitochondria are the major site of reactive oxygen species (ROS) production in the cell; therefore, it is likely that progressive decline in mitochondrial function is due to the accumulation of oxidative damage with age."

In a paper titled "Oxidative stress and mitochondrial dysfunction in neurodegenerative diseases," E. Trushina and C. T. McMurray showed that reactive oxygen species, typically generated from mitochondrial respiration, cause oxidative damage of nucleic acids, lipids, carbohydrates and proteins. [13] Despite enormous effort, however, the mechanism by which oxidative damage causes neuronal death is not well understood. Emerging data from a number of neuro-degenerative diseases suggest that there may be common features of toxicity that are related to oxidative damage.

Aleksandra Trifunovic and her colleagues at the Karolinska Institute in Sweden, genetically engineered a line of mice to carry a compromised version of an enzyme, which normally proofreads mitochondrial DNA to ensure proper replication and repair.[14] The use of such transgenic animals is becoming increasingly common in studies of aging and disease.

Trifunovic found that subsequent tests of the brain, heart and liver cells of their mice revealed three to five times more errors in their mitochondrial DNA as found in normal mice. By twenty-five weeks of age, these mutants began to develop the usual signs of aging for mice, including chronic diseases much like those seen in humans. None of them lived as long as their littermate controls. Now we find that statin drugs are similarly compromising our mitochondrial failsafe measures.

Meanwhile, mitochondrial impairment is increasingly implicated in the side effects of statins, and even the side effects of other commonly used drugs. Nadanaciva, S., and others, examined rat liver mitochondria to determine the effects of six different statin drugs and several drugs commonly used in the treatment of type 2 diabetes. [15] They were using special techniques to study the mitochondrial process of oxidative phosphorylation (OXPHOS), key to energy formation in the body. They found that all statins impaired the enzymes vital to this OXPHOS process, some far more than others, but in addition found that commonly used type 2 diabetes medications were potent inhibitors of this process as well.

Obviously, the combination of both statins and type 2 diabetes drugs yielded the greatest effects on mitochondrial mutations. Needless to say, the authors of this study were careful to avoid disparaging specific drugs to avoid undue concern by patients under treatment, but the bottom line is that all statin drugs cause mitochondrial damage in our energy equation, and if you are being treated for type 2 diabetes as well, the likelihood of significant damage is even greater.

Recently, the volume of research on this subject is increasing rapidly as scientists explore possible treatment options for minimizing the effects of reactive oxygen species damage, and for modulating mitochondrial mutations. Most of these studies are being done with natural product supplements.

Natural product selection depends upon a careful analysis of each component and biochemical reactions in the energy equation. All of these are now well known. The major players are CoQ10 and vitamins B3 and B2 (also known as NADH and FADH2 or niacin and riboflavin). Most people have not the slightest awareness of the important roles of these three common substances. And it is the same in all organisms. Even our most basic organisms, billions of years into the past, had this system of energy. It was so good that Mother Nature found no reason to change during the long process of evolution.

Almost every cell in our bodies is able to convert glucose into energy in the form of adenosine triphosphate, or ATP. ATP contains high-energy phosphate bonds, which, when broken, release energy that drives the various chemical processes for any particular cell.

The process of creating energy from glucose occurs in two ways: the first way (called glycolysis) does not make much energy and does not require oxygen or many nutrients. The second way (called oxidation) creates much more energy – but this requires B-vitamins, minerals, lots of CoQ10, and the presence of oxygen. In healthy cells, glycolysis can only make 10% of the available energy from glucose – but oxidation can extract the remaining 90% of available energy from glucose. Again, oxidation requires the presence of CoQ10.

References for:
Mitochondrial Damage in Aging

1. Vladutiu, G. and others. Statin associated myopathy with normal CK levels. *Ann Int Med* 137; 581-86, 2002

2. Rifai, Z. Ragged Red fibers in normal aging and inflammatory myopathy. *Neuro* 37; 24-29, 1995

3. Carvalho, J. and others. Statins and fibrates associated myopathy: study of eight cases. *Arch Neuro Psych* 62, No 2a, 2003

4. Nicolson and Ellithorpe. Lipid Replacement and Antioxidant Nutritional Therapy for Restoring Mitochondrial Function and

Reducing Fatigue in Chronic Fatigue Syndrome and other Fatiguing Illnesses. *Journal of Chronic Fatigue Syndrome* 13(1): 57-68, 2006

5. Huang and Manton. Role of oxidative damage in mitochondria during aging. *Frontiers in Bioscience* 9:1100-1117, 2004

6. Brierly, E. J. and others. Mitochondrial mutations in the elderly. *Annals of Neurology* 43(2) 217-23, 2004

7. Wei and Lee. Oxidative Stress, Mitochondrial DNA Mutation, and Impairment of Antioxidant Enzymes in Aging. *Exp Biol and Med* 227:671-682, 2002

8. Halliwell, B. Role of free radicals in neurodegenerative diseases: therapeutic implications for antioxidant treatment. *Drugs Aging* 18:685-716, 2001

9. Xu and Finkel. Role for mitochondria as potential regulators of cellular life span. *Biochem Biophysics Res Commun* 294:245-248, 2002

10. Lin and others. High aggregate burden of somatic mitochondrial DNA point mutations, in aging and Alzheimer's disease brains. *Human Molecular Genetics* 11: 133-45, 2002.

11. Nojiri, N. and others. Oxidative stress causes heart failure with impaired mitochondrial respiration. *J Biol Chem* 281; 33789-801, 2006

12. Singh, K. Mitochondria Damage Checkpoint, Aging, and Cancer. *Annals of New York Academy of Sciences* 1067; 182-90, 2006

13. Trushina, E. and McMurray, C. Oxidative stress and mitochondrial dysfunction in neurodegenerative diseases. *Neuroscience* 145; 44: 1233-48, 2007

14. Trifunovic, A. Does premature aging of the mtDNA mutator mouse prove that mtDNA mutations are involved in natural aging? *Aging Cell* 5 (3) 279-82, 2007

15. Nadanaciva, S. and others. Current Concepts in Drug Induced Mitochondrial Toxicity. *Toxicol Appl Pharmacol.* May, 2009

Mitochondrial Damage in Aging
Chapter Summary and Key Points.

- Statin use has been linked to myopathy, without muscle enzyme abnormality.

- With a lack of availability of sufficient CoQ10 and glutathione, rapid mitochondrial mutation can be expected.

- Oxidative damage is implicated in many human age-related diseases.

- With age, mitochondrial function declines and mitochondrial DNA (mtDNA) mutations increase.

- Studies show that mtDNA abnormalities are involved in the aging process in human muscle.

- In diseases such as Alzheimer's, oxidative stress and oxidative damage is felt to play a key role in the loss of neurons, and the progression to dementia.

- Mitochondrial impairment is increasingly implicated in the side effects of statins.

- In a study, the combination of statins and type 2 diabetes drugs yielded the greatest effects on mitochondrial mutations.

- The oxidation process of making energy requires vitamins B3 and B2, minerals, lots of CoQ10, and the presence of oxygen.

Mitochondrial Mutations and Dietary Supplements

Relevant to statin damage, we have recently learned much about natural causes of mitochondrial damage. Studies of chronic fatigue and other infirmities of age have documented the progressive loss of the ability of mitochondria to produce high-energy molecules (ATP) for cell function. We now know that progressive damage to our mitochondria results from exposure to the so-called free radicals. These highly reactive oxygen species (ROS), inevitably lead to modifications of mitochondrial lipids, proteins and DNA, known as mutations, and are a consequence of natural aging.

Ordinarily, our antioxidant system is sufficient to overcome this daily oxidative stress, but due to the combination of our predetermined genetic make-up, nutrition factors and exposure to disease, our anti-oxidation capacity, never 100% in its effectiveness, gradually deteriorates as we age. This allows excess build-up of ROS, the primary cause of the mitochondrial damage or mutations that accumulate as we age.

This knowledge has supported a huge research effort directed at the use of nutritional supplements, in an attempt to bolster failing metabolic and anti-oxidation systems. Every aspect of the human energy equation has been looked at, and thousands of research studies have been conducted to determine possible benefits from supplementing with many vital substances of oxidative phosphorylation and anti-oxidation pathways.

Now we find that among the many side effects of statin drug use, is the same direct assault on our mitochondrial DNA, and our energy equation, produced by natural aging.

The well-known statin side effect of coenzyme Q10 inhibition, bears directly upon the effectiveness of our anti-oxidation system, leading directly to excess ROS production, with its age-like mutagenic consequences.

Additionally, another well-known statin side effect — that of dolichol inhibition — results directly in failure of glycoprotein synthesis. This leads to a loss of effectiveness of many of our glycoprotein based systems, such as glycohydrolases, for detection and correction of DNA damage. Statin drugs cause effects on our mitochondria identical to those that accumulate with age. One might say that one side effect of statin therapy is premature aging.

My research over the years has slowly revealed the various mechanisms of action of statin drugs in the production of side effects. First, I learned about statin drug inhibition of glial cell cholesterol, so vital for memory. Then on the basis of detailed study of the inevitable statin associated mevalonate blockade of CoQ10 and dolichol synthesis, I learned about the consequent neuropathies, myopathies and chronic neuromuscular degeneration.

Now I know why many of the statin side effects are permanent and why weakness and fatigue are such common complaints. Many statin victims say that abruptly, almost in the blink of an eye, they have become old people. Doctors, for the most part unaware of the truth, reassuringly say, "You have to expect these things now at your age. You are not thirty anymore." Unwittingly, doctors have come close to the mark, for aging is what statins do.

Treatment of this effect of statins must involve all that nutritional researchers have learned these past few years in their quest for youth. Currently, there is no conventional medical, or pharmaceutical treatment, for the prevention and treatment of mitochondrial mutations. However, everything that nutritional researchers consider useful and appropriate for fatigue and aging therapy, may also be relevant for statin damage. The list of substances found to be relevant to the process of oxidative phosphorylation and anti-oxidation in the human body, is extensive.

Antioxidants found useful: vitamin C, vitamin E (tocotrienols and tocopherols), coenzyme Q10, alpha-lipoic acid, N-acetyl cysteine, carotenoids, flavonoids and many others.

Important accessory molecules include vitamin B3 (niacin), vitamin B6 (pyridoxine hydrochloride), vitamin B12 (cyanocobalamin), vitamin B2 (riboflavin), folic acid (folate), melatonin, magnesium, selenium, zinc, phosphatidylcholine, and related compounds.

There is no way the average person can look at this list and formulate his or her personal requirements for mitochondrial repair. Even medical professionals, after a lifetime of experience, must work hard to convert these elements of metabolism and anti-oxidation into a rational plan for help.

Although we have the technological ability to measure the various components of our electron transport, oxidative phosphorylation and beta-oxidative systems, the cost of doing so would be prohibitive; the only rational approach appears to be the administration of supplements, on a broad spectrum basis, with critical appraisal of the response.

I have taken on the task of selecting from this list of available supplements, those that impress me most with their potential to help slow down or reverse this process of statin-associated mitochondrial mutations. I will present each one without regard for relative effect.

CoQ10: I consider CoQ10 to be critical for mitochondrial maintenance. Not only is it a powerful antioxidant, superbly located to protect our mitochondria from oxidative damage, but also, as an integral part of the energy producing complexes of the mitochondria, it is key to electron transport and ATP production. Our ability to synthesize CoQ10 falls off with age and after maturity, we are almost completely dependent upon diet or supplements, and diets are frequently deficient.

Vitamin C: Vitamin C is a powerful antioxidant with many essential roles in the body. The only argument one might have with the U.S. government's Recommended Daily Intake (RDI), is that all the many roles of vitamin C have not been accounted for. The current RDI, is only sufficient to prevent death or serious health issues from acute deficiency of vitamin C (e.g., scurvy). The RDI is also adequate for required collagen and hormone synthesis (the RDI is mainly based on this). But to work effectively as an antioxidant, scientists are learning that vitamin C levels need to be significantly higher in our bodies.

The debate now is over how much is needed. The Tolerable Upper Intake Level (UL), is the maximum continual intake of a nutrient that is unlikely to cause adverse health effects in almost all people — for vitamin C, this has been defined as 2 grams per day (2,000 mg/day) in divided doses.

Selenium: The predominant biochemical action of selenium in humans is to serve as an antioxidant via the selenium-dependent enzyme, glutathione peroxidase, and thus protect cellular membranes and organelles from peroxidative damage.

Without sufficient selenium, you must expect both reduced cellular energy from adenosine triphosphate (ATP) and increased mitochondrial damage from reactive oxygen species (ROS).

The use of statin drugs has served to increase attention on the role of selenoproteins in humans, as statins tend to block the vital mevalonate pathway by which selenoproteins are utilized.

To date, well over 30 selenoprotein enzymes have been discovered for the element selenium, expressing an unusually wide range of physiological applications with multi-system involvement. These enzymes are highly beneficial in preventing mitochondrial damage, premature aging, and many chronic diseases — similar to the antioxidant role of CoQ10.

There is also evidence that selenium has a protective effect against some forms of cancer, and that it may decrease cardiovascular disease mortality, and be essential for a healthy immune response.

In summary, selenium has critical roles in mitochondrial maintenance, muscular metabolism and brain function, and is vital in general metabolism and thyroid function, but we are only just beginning to make informed assessments.

100mcg to 200mcg of selenium as a daily requirement for an average adult impresses me as being a reasonable amount. Caution, though, should be exercised when supplementing with selenium. Although selenium is essential for good health, too much is just as bad as too little. Selenium toxicity can occur with amounts over 400 micrograms daily for adults.

Regular consumption of foods that contain selenium can easily meet daily requirements. Brazil nuts are a particularly rich source of selenium, and just one or two per day can keep body selenium at its optimum level.[1] Other dietary sources of selenium are sunflower seeds, fish, red meat, poultry, eggs and onions.

Lecithin: Of the tens of thousands of molecules that make up the life of a cell, phosphatidylcholine stands apart as the major component of the membrane — the structural skin that surrounds the cell as well as the tiny organelles within it.

But it is far more than an outside protective layer. With this vital membrane, PUFAs (polyunsaturated fatty acids) form the essence of life function. Cellular membranes are bi-lipid layers of opposing phospholipids lined up, soldier-fashion, that automatically organize themselves into a spherical shape to provide the protecting outer cover. Within this membrane sits a huge selection of ion channels and receptors, from a genetic library, that literally run the entire system. It is very important to take capsules or granules at fully recommended doses.

Omega-3 & 6 (essential fatty acids): Essential fatty acids cannot be synthesized by the body so requirements must come from the diet or dietary supplements.

Much has recently been learned about omega-3 & 6, also known as PUFAs and their importance, even necessity, in mitochondrial maintenance. Until recently, the typical western diet had become relatively high in omega-6 and relatively low in omega-3 fatty acids, thus the emphasis for supplementation has been almost exclusively on omega-3.

Now, however, due to extensive food processing in the modern world, we find that much of the ingested omega-6 has been inactive. This occurs due to the routine penning of animals used for eggs and meat, plus modern food preservation, processing, storage and cooking. Animals raised in such a fashion and the foods derived, are deficient both in the amount and in the proper balance of the essential fatty acids — omega-3 to omega-6. Omega balance is the key to proper metabolism.[2]

D-Ribose: Studies indicate that oral consumption of D-Ribose leads to increased power productivity and improves the capacity of skeletal muscles to quickly recover energy levels. Our ATP levels decrease during exercise and normally take considerable time to recover. Even after days of rest, research shows that without supplementation, skeletal muscle has a limited ability to maintain peak performance during periods of repetitive high intensity exercise.

High levels of cellular energy are required to keep tissues running at peak performance. D-Ribose has also been used to reduce fatigue in chronic fatigue syndrome. Another interesting feature of this sugar supplement is that it comprises the backbone of ribonucleic acid (RNA), the basis of our genetic transcription and, through the removal of one hydroxyl group, becomes deoxyribonucleic acid (DNA). Because of this, it is a promising element in any attempt to repair DNA damage.

Tocotrienols, Vitamin E: Tocotrienols are the new and much improved form of the vitamin E family.[3] Supplemental vitamin E needs these past decades have been almost exclusively met by tocopherols, especially alpha-tocopherol, and it is tocotrienol poor.

Tocotrienols increase CoQ10 and dolichols, thereby helping greatly to offset the inhibitory effects of mevalonate blockade. Tocotrienols directly inhibit reactive oxygen species (ROS) and in combination with CoQ10, help quench ROS better. Tocotrienols mimic the anti-inflammatory effects of statins in their inhibition of platelet aggregation and activation, while at the same time reducing monocyte adhesion and macrophage recruitment — the primary elements of the inflammatory response — thereby reducing cardiovascular risk, without the penalty of mevalonate blockade.

This combination of effects serves to reduce both lipid oxidation as well as mitochondrial DNA damage. Tocotrienols also have a 50% greater effectiveness as an antioxidant than the tocopherol form of vitamin E, making them even more desirable for mitochondrial maintenance purposes. Both tocotrienols and CoQ10 are isoprenoids, with tocotrienol working exogenously and CoQ10 working endogenously, to bring maximum antioxidant benefit to the cell membrane surface.

Magnesium: The average American consumes only 40% of the recommended daily allowance of magnesium. Magnesium activates 76% of the enzymes in the body, and many of these enzymes are in our mitochondrial energy equation. Without enough "biologically available" magnesium, the cellular calcium pump slows down. Therefore, low levels of available magnesium inhibit the generation of energy. The end result is that the mitochondrion, which is the powerhouse of the cell and the entire body, degenerates.

L-carnitine: The adult form of carnitine palmitoyltransferase (CPT) II deficiency has been labeled as the most common lipid myopathy in humans. This autosomal, recessively inherited disease, may be even more prevalent than generally believed due to under-recognition of the disorder.[4, 5]

CPT II is associated with the inner mitochondrial membrane. It works together with carnitine-acylcarnitine translocase, an inner mitochondrial membrane enzyme, to facilitate the transport of lipids (fatty acids) across these membranes and into the mitochondrial matrix, where they are ultimately converted to energy in the form of ATP.

Extremely important in many people, and you never know who needs it.

Alpha-Lipoic Acid (ALA): ALA is a vital coenzyme in the mitochondria's Krebs cycle for the production of cellular energy. It directly recycles and extends the metabolic lifespans of vitamin C, glutathione, vitamin E and coenzyme Q10. Since coenzyme Q10 is of major importance to the mitochondrial electron transport chain, this effect of ALA is particularly beneficial. In the United States, it is sold as a dietary supplement, usually as 50 mg tablets. Note that ALA also enhances the effect of other supplemental antioxidants.

Vitamin D: Only in the last ten to fifteen years has the powerful role in anti-inflammation been recognized for vitamin D. It is also known as calcitriol — the hormonally active part of vitamin D. For the previous 50 years, we knew only of its critical role in the regulation of calcium in our bodies and of bone metabolism. I suspect there is still more yet to come from current research on vitamin D.

Recently, an impressive body of work shows that calcitriol also acts as an anti-inflammatory agent that functions by influencing immune cell interactions. For example, different subtypes of immune cells communicate by secreting factors called cytokines to initiate a particular type of immune response. Vitamin D has been shown to repress exaggerated inflammatory responses by inhibiting that cytokine cross-talk. Plentiful animal research has served to corroborate this.

A possible role of vitamin D in reducing the effects of excessive oxidation on our mitochondria must be considered. Recent studies suggest that no less than half of U.S. adults need to consume at least 1,000 IU of vitamin D3 daily or to generate it in the skin by exposure to sunlight.

Pyrroloquinoline quinone (PQQ): A few years ago, I learned of another biochemical that is also implicated in the process of mitochondrial maintenance. The name of this substance is pyrroloquinoline quinone (PQQ).

The vital role of PQQ in mitochondrial support has only been documented in the past fifteen years. From what I have read of this substance, it is worth considering for those of us who have been damaged by statins, whether by cognitive dysfunction, permanent myopathy, ALS-like symptoms, or peripheral neuropathy.

Dietary sources of PQQ include many fruits and vegetables and egg yolk. Natto (fermented soybeans), is a particularly rich source as are celery, parsley, papaya and kiwi fruit. PQQ is also available as a dietary supplement. Human trials and studies will need to be performed to support any claims for the benefits of PQQ supplementation. One promotion for PQQ begins with, "The more functional mitochondria you have in your cells, the greater your overall health and durability," which is the premise of this book, so my interest in this substance is obvious.

The problem is that as we age, our mitochondria degrade and become dysfunctional. Compared with nuclear DNA, mitochondrial DNA is left almost entirely exposed to the ravages of free radicals. It attaches directly to the inner membrane where the mitochondria's furnace rages continuously.

Statin drugs directly hasten this process of mitochondrial DNA degradation by direct inhibition of CoQ10 and dolichol synthesis. The ultimate cause of statin associated adverse reactions, is this progressive deterioration of mitochondrial DNA. PQQ is being touted not only for its extra antioxidant protection in the fight against free radicals, but also for its potential use for mitochondrial genesis.

The challenge aging humans face is that methods to increase the generation of new mitochondria are difficult to adhere to. Up until recently, the only natural ways to stimulate mitochondrial genesis were calorie restriction or exhaustive physical activity. You may have heard of the half-starved mice that were run to exhaustion, and most share the opinion that this research, though interesting, is not applicable to humans. However, PQQ research has shown some very interesting results. Experimental animals deprived of PQQ, in addition to stunted growth and development, reveal fewer mitochondria in their tissues. When PQQ is restored, normal growth and development return, and the mitochondrial number is increased.

This has led researchers to the effect of PQQ on certain genes having to do with control of the process of mitochondrial genesis. Their work has led to the promising idea that we now may be able to trigger mitochondrial genesis through the use of this dietary supplement. This seems almost too good to be true, but at this time I cannot fault the research results, and feel comfortable in at least bringing it to the attention of statin damage victims and their doctors.

When one compares the boundless energy of a child with the slow shuffle of a senior citizen, it is easy to understand the impact of our mitochondria. Mitochondria in the muscles of a child, are nearly all burning hot with available energy, whereas studies have revealed that in the muscles of seniors, some 95% of their mitochondria is damaged — their once energetic powerhouses have now gone cold.

Many things contribute to the maintenance and function of mitochondria. The biochemical processes that we have evolved to derive our energy needs are remarkably tolerant, permitting us to more or less cover this planet of ours despite widely varying diets.

Just as we have recently discovered the adverse effect of statin drugs on mitochondrial DNA, now we have discovered still another substance vital to mitochondrial function. Not only does PQQ appear to bring us enhanced anti-oxidation to help fight the constant war against free radicals, it also offers the possibility of mitochondrial growth.

Research support for this new concept of mitochondrial genesis is rapidly accumulating. In January 2010, Lanza and Nair of the Mayo Clinic, using liver cells, showed in experimental animals that the influence of PQQ is on the pathways that previous research has shown to regulate mitochondrial biogenesis.[6]

This extraordinary work on mitochondrial function was confirmed by Chowanadisai and others at the University of California, Davis.

Tao and others of the San Francisco VA Medical Center and The University of California, San Francisco (UCSF), used adult rat heart cells to demonstrate the ability of PQQ to preserve mitochondrial function and prevent oxidative injury.[7]

Thus solid evidence exists for the role of PQQ in both liver and heart cells and almost undoubtedly further research will demonstrate a similar effect in any tissue studied, for mitochondrial function is not tissue specific.

References for:
Mitochondrial Mutations and Dietary Supplements

1. Ref: https://www.ncbi.nlm.nih.gov/pubmed/18258628

2. Peskin, B. and Habib, A. *The hidden story of Cancer*, Pinnacle Press, 2008

3. Tan, B. and Mueller, A. *Tocotrienols*: *Vitamin E beyond Tocopherol*. Watson, R. AOCS Press, 2008

4. Vladutiu, G. and others. Genetic risk factors associated with lipid-lowering drug-induced myopathies. *Muscle Nerve* 34(2):153-62, 2006

5. Vladutiu, G. Genetic predisposition to statin myopathy. *Curr Opin Rheumatol* 20:648-655, 2008

6. *Pflugers Archives*, 459(2); 277-89, January 2010, Lanza and Nair of the Mayo Clinic

7. Tao et al. Biochem Biophys Res Commun. 16;363(2):257-62. Nov. 2007.

Mitochondrial Mutations and Dietary Supplements
Chapter Summary and Key Points.

- Studies of chronic fatigue show the progressive loss of the ability of mitochondria to produce high-energy molecules for cell function.

- Our anti-oxidation capacity gradually deteriorates as we age.

- Among the many side effects of statins is the same direct assault on our mitochondrial DNA produced by natural aging.

- One side effect of statin therapy is premature aging.

- Currently, there is no conventional medical, or pharmaceutical treatment for the prevention and treatment of mitochondrial mutations.

- What is considered useful and appropriate for fatigue and aging therapy by nutritional researchers, may also be relevant for statin damage.

- CoQ10 is critical for mitochondrial maintenance as an anti-oxidant and as part of the energy producing complexes.

- Vitamin C is a powerful antioxidant at higher doses than the RDI, which is beneficial only in preventing scurvy, and maintaining collagen and hormone synthesis.

- Selenium is an antioxidant that has critical roles in mitochondrial maintenance, muscular metabolism and brain function, and is vital in general metabolism and thyroid function. Selenium toxicity can occur with amounts over 400 micrograms daily for adults.

- Lecithin is a major component of the membrane of cells.

- Omega-3 & 6 (Essential Fatty Acids): Essential fatty acids cannot be synthesized by the body so requirements must come from the diet or dietary supplements.

- D-Ribose improves the capacity of skeletal muscles to recover after exercise.

- Tocotrienols increase CoQ10 and dolichols and mimic the anti-inflammatory effects of statins.

- Magnesium activates 76% of the enzymes in the body.

- Alpha-lipoic acid directly recycles and extends the metabolic lifespans of vitamin C, glutathione, vitamin E and coenzyme Q10.

- Pyrroloquinoline quinone is being touted not only for its extra antioxidant protection in the fight against free radicals, but also for its potential use for mitochondrial growth.

Mitochondrial Mutations: Diet

One of the first considerations in any plan for mitochondrial maintenance should be a hard look at dietary intake. There is much you can do to optimize the ability of your body for self-repair, and that ability extends also to the mitochondria.

In the previous chapter on supplements, I referred to a number of vitamins and minerals that we know are intimately involved in mitochondrial formation and function. Eight amino acids are generally regarded as essential for adult humans. Four others are also essential for infants and growing children. In addition, certain amino acids are considered "conditionally essential," meaning they are not normally required in the diet, but must be added for certain people who are genetically deficient in their ability to synthesize them.

The ability of the human body to adapt is truly amazing. Many of these specific essential needs have only recently been identified. In the case of polyunsaturated fatty acids (PUFAs), the fact that omega-3 was essential to our diet was learned relatively recently, and the role of the omegas in cell wall and mitochondrial membrane construction has made the omegas particularly relevant to mitochondrial repair and maintenance; and still we are learning. Personally, I am amazed at how much we have learned since I graduated from medical school, and I marvel at the speed at which new information is accumulating.

Much has happened to our diets since our Paleolithic days that ended 10,000 years ago. However, applying the customary time scale for genetic change, our bodies and our metabolic functions are virtually the same as they were when our ancestors gave up the hunter-gatherer existence.

For 45,000 years, the usual estimate for the emergence of modern man, the Paleolithic diet served us well. During 25,000 of these years, ancestors for many of us co-existed with our Neanderthal cousins who had lived the same hunter-gatherer lifestyle for over 200,000 years. Two million years earlier, Australopithecus (early humans), had lived a very similar hunter-gatherer life in Africa.

As evidenced by archeological finds of robust skeletal remains and healthy teeth, the Homo sapiens' diet was well suited for this phase of life. Any pathologist on looking over fossil remains from that era, would conclude a relative absence of diseases, and generally healthy specimens. Fine teeth and strong bones testify to adequate nutrition.

As nutritional opportunists, we have easily adjusted to diets radically different from our past. However, the question remains. What is the ideal diet for humans, the diet to which they are optimally adapted? In my judgment there is but one answer, that the nutritional needs of our bodies are still best met by the foodstuffs consumed during our hunter-gatherer phase of existence.

The diet of our pre-agricultural ancestors consisted of meats, insects, eggs, plants, roots, tubers, fruits, seeds and nuts. Meats should be further defined to include the flesh of water creatures, such as fish and shellfish, as well as the flesh of animals. Of course, such variety was restricted by both seasonal and geographical factors.

Much insight about this subject of hunter-gatherer existence has come from the study of small pockets of aboriginals still living the life of their forefathers, such as the Bushmen of Botswana, more commonly known as the Kung San of the Kalahari, and the Inuit of Greenland. In both of these groups, their nutrition over the past few decades has rapidly changed in response to increasing contact with governmental agencies, missionaries, and even well-meaning anthropologists, so that today these few pockets of Paleolithic life no longer exist in pure form.

The Kung San tribe has been particularly illustrative in defining just how a primitive group goes about the process of living off the land. The evolving picture comes very close to what our remote ancestors must have faced in Africa, hundreds of thousands of years ago, and represents a system of life well tested.

Anthropologist Richard Lee has studied the nutritional needs of the Kung San for a long time.[1] He maintains that the security of their life is attributable mainly to the fact that vegetables, not meat, form the mainstay of their diet. Plant foods are abundant, locally available, and predictable. Game animals, in contrast, are scarce and unpredictable.

In addition to the mongongo nut, they have an astonishing availability of 105 edible plants: 14 fruits and nuts, 15 berries, 18 species of edible gum, 41 edible roots and bulbs and 17 leafy greens, melons, and other foods. Meat contributes 30 percent of the calories to the diet, and hunting was the major occupation of the men.

The other side of the coin for permanently living off the land is one of settlement patterns. Diet and mobility must go hand in hand, for sooner or later every settlement must be nearly exhausted of mongongo nuts, game, water or other critical dietary items, forcing the moving on of the tribe to more productive areas.

Ultimately, a seasonal pattern of movement evolves wherever primitive man existed, governed by such factors as water supply, game movement or availability of key foodstuffs. The Kung San have developed a system of well-built seasonal shelters, inhabited for several months each year, along with their use of portable "traveling shelters" suitable for use for shorter time periods, in which the structural poles can be bundled together and carried.

This pattern of life met the needs of Paleolithic man for tens of thousands of years, and can be adapted to any reasonable climate and temperature range. For groups having access to large bodies of water, where subsistence is constantly available, settlement patterns become of relatively minor importance. Such sites may well have been the models for permanent settlements, fostering the introduction and increased dependency of agriculture to come.

I dwell on these few remaining vestiges of Paleolithic hunter-gatherer life to illustrate how well it has served mankind, and how ingrained our physiology is to this thoroughly tested cultural pattern from our ancestors.

I would like now to introduce the Inuit of Greenland to illustrate the frequently observed motto, "you are what you eat." Susan Allport, medical journalist, has done an excellent job of expressing the importance of what we eat in her book, *The Queen of Fats*.[2] In putting this book together, she has introduced us to dozens of research scientists, and their contributions to our underlying dietary needs.

Her story starts with the Greenland Inuit, and their relative absence of heart disease. This group is a remnant of Paleolithic man who, instead of remaining in Africa, as did the Kung San, migrated across Europe, and eventually the Bering Strait 12,000 years ago. This was the original filling of the Americas with man, with this group settling in the far north, adapting to the climatic condition of cold and ice, just as the Kung San had adapted to heat and aridity.

What we have learned from these Inuit is nothing short of amazing. Thankfully, it has kept the scientific community focused on fats for years. The diet of the Inuit is essentially fish and seal meat. Despite this heavy focus on fat, their blood fat measurements were found to be remarkably normal when compared to a control population of Copenhagen citizens.

The Inuit did not differ at all in blood cholesterol, triglycerides, LDL cholesterol, VLDL cholesterol — all the usual parameters — except for their HDLs, which were very elevated. In addition, their bleeding times were found to be some 8 minutes, twice the generally accepted normal value.

They had mentioned frequent nosebleeds in their history, but not as a problem, only as an observation. As to their heart disease deaths, the strokes and heart attacks common to our society back in the early seventies, they had almost none. This was a subject demanding of study, and only with the availability of special equipment did the truths finally emerge.

This had to do with PUFAs, polyunsaturated fatty acids. This was when we were made aware of the difference between the omega-3 fats, those of alpha linolenic acid, and omega-6 fats, linoleic acid. For the first time, we learned that both are essential to our diet, and therefore must be consumed in proper balance.

Omega-3 PUFAs have two common derivatives — DHA, docosahexaenoic acid, and EPA, eicosapentaenoic acid. The blood samples of the Inuit were loaded with EPAs, and their primary diet of fish and seal was also loaded with EPAs. Yes, they had other fats such as DHA derivatives, but it was the EPA values that were notably elevated.

The scientist ultimately found that the fatty acids of the food consumed by the Inuit became the fatty acids in their bodies, so important to such physiologic functions as platelet activation and blood clotting. These people as a group were bleeders, not clotters, but one usually does not die of bleeding. Nosebleeds once or twice a week are a nuisance, but you don't die of them. It is the clotters who die, of strokes and heart attacks.

We learned much about physiology during the research on PUFAs. They are the substance of membranes and cell walls. Their job is to create membranes, so delicate and porous, you hardly know they are there. Somehow, it has to hold in or keep out specific substances, yet allow instantaneous entry and exit of other vital substances.

It is unapparent and inconsequential — hardly more than water itself. That is the job of our omegas, twenty carbons in length and pure magic in function, and the most magical of all is DHA. It is the fatty acid closest in liquidity to pure water, allowing almost instantaneous reactions so that it expedites cellular reactions of all kinds.

The greatest concentration of it is in our brains and eyes. Need I also add that DHA content correlated directly with metabolic rate and activity? Highly active, short-lived creatures have high levels of DHA. Large, slow and long-lived creatures have low DHA values.

These same magic fats, in proper ratios between omega-3 and omega-6, actually shifted the balance of coagulation factors in the Inuit to anti-coagulation. This encouraged at least one Oxford don (tutor) to eat seal meat every day for a year, and with this information in the media, the resulting boom in the sale of fish oil capsules occurred almost everywhere.

It seems that in our natural Paleolithic state, our dietary intake of omega-6 to omega-3 was about even at 1:1. Since that time, however, there has been a gradual trend for omega-6 intake to increase relative to omega-3 — at first, simply because of the changing character of our foodstuffs.

In the past 100 years or so, other factors such as food preservation and processing measures have gradually diminished omega-3 because its unsaturated state makes it far more sensitive to oxidative change. The ratio now is estimated by various authorities to be 10, 20, or even 30:1, compared to the 1:1 of our hunter-gatherer era.

Even more recently, in the past 30 years or so, chickens and cattle are only free-ranging from specialist farms. The vast majority are pen-raised. It is now almost impossible to make an accurate estimate of the omega-6:3 ratio since both omega-6 and 3 are nutritionally threatened by pen-raising and corn feeding. The eggs of penned chickens and the meat of pen-raised animals are radically different in omega content, especially omega-6.

PUFAs are sleepers, in the sense that we are only now beginning to appreciate just how powerful the effects are on our bodies from deficiencies or imbalance of these dietary fats. I remember the first time, during World War II, when I got a bag of solid fat with a little yellow tab inside. You broke the tab and squeezed the bag and there it was — butter substitute, or should I say, margarine.

Few of us realized the true health implication of this, except for Paul Dudley White, cardiologist to President Eisenhower in 1955 while I was at Walter Reed Hospital. He knew the health implications and publicly refused to get on the cholesterol bandwagon. The entire food marketing, drug industry and medical world immediately turned their collective backs to him.

I still remember his words of warning about corn oil. They went something like this "I hung up my shingle as a cardiologist in 1921 and had to wait until 1928 to get my first referral for a heart attack. Then came the war and margarine and the drastic change in our diet. Corn oil is the cause."

Gone was real butter and lard. In their place was a never ending stream of substitutes, all of them alien to our diets, along with a never ending stream of heart attacks and strokes. We have learned so much about PUFAs in just the past four decades. Now we know they are intimately involved in cancer proneness, cardiac arrhythmias of all kinds, and even behavioral and emotional problems.

All this is now being taught in medical school, long after I graduated. I had practiced medicine for years, not even knowing that PUFAs like omega-3 and 6 are essential, and having no idea of the possible negative impact of the food industry on their availability in our daily diet. Something so vital it can substitute for statin drugs, and I have only recently learned of it — and from a medical writer, not from my extensive medical training program.

I strongly recommend reading *The Queen of Fats* by Susan Allport for greater detail into this important subject. Only a medical journalist could have summarized the thoughts of so many of the principal lipid investigators so well. In addition, she has touched my heart with one of her final statements: "Recommendations to reduce dietary cholesterol and [the use of statins to] block the synthesis of cholesterol, a necessary component of brain function, will one day seem as quaint as bloodletting."

Those of you who have followed my long-running opposition to the war on cholesterol, and the mind-robbing potential of statin drugs, will understand completely my pleasure to read this in her book.

In his forward thinking diet book, *The Heart Revolution*, Kilmer McCully, M.D. reviewed the many ramifications of a diet that supports his concept of elevated homocysteine playing a major role in arterial inflammation. Homocysteine appears to be the primary trigger of atherosclerosis in at least 40% of cases, according to Dr. McCully.

Other factors such as oxycholesterol, trans fats, improper omega-3:6 ratios, smoking and hidden infections are likely causative in most of the remainder. In addition, a subset of individuals may have inherited coagulation and platelet factors that predispose them to atherosclerosis.

Dr. McCully tells us that folic acid (B9), and vitamins B6 and B12 have vital contributions to the proper metabolism of homocysteine, and that their deficiencies will lead to an excess of homocysteine.

Some people are born with deficiencies of one or the other of these three B vitamins, resulting in early death from arterial damage, which leads to strokes and heart attacks. It was the reality of children with elevated homocysteine levels dying at age five and six of stroke, heart failure and kidney failure that led Dr. McCully to his discovery of homocysteine elevation as the cause.

Dr. McCully also examined the food storage and processing factors that can contribute to deficiencies in these B vitamins and their vital co-factors. Many vitamins, including the B complex, are often unable to function without adequate amounts of minerals such as zinc, magnesium, silicon and copper, and even other vitamins.

These critical co-factors may often be made deficient in foods by improper storage and processing procedures. McCully counsels the best way to eat food is in its simplest form. Fruits should be eaten raw as much as possible. Vegetables that cannot be eaten raw should be steamed, with minimal water, or briefly stir-fried. Avoid the prolonged heat exposure of boiling or deep-fat frying.

Avoid canning. Freeze for storage. Do not overcook. These guidelines will give you optimal preservation of B6 and folic acid. B12 is much more stable and tolerant of heat. The same cooking and storage rules generally apply to meats. Light grilling and broiling is always best.

The key to proper eating, according to McCully, "Is to cut out the processed, packaged, fast foods devoid of nutrients, and focus on eating fresh, whole, unprocessed foods."

Essentially, without saying it, McCully is advising us to return closer to our old Paleolithic diet; the diet our ancestors consumed for hundreds of thousands of years before we settled down in small agrarian communities.

Our civilized diet that has come with cultivation, our grain crops and more recently sugar, are anomalies. But that does not mean we cannot forage and eat like our hunter-gatherer ancestors — it just means we have to confine our hunting and gathering to supermarkets.

There are dozens of diet books out there that can satisfy specific, even eccentric demands. The diet Dr. McCully is talking about is definitely protein augmented and carbohydrate restrictive, and that being said, it is a fine, healthy way to eat. When I say "carbo-restrictive", I am talking of the refined carbohydrates — the sugars, white breads and white rice types of foodstuffs, almost completely devoid of all but calories.

His protein sources do include beans, nuts, soybeans and lentils, but he reminds us that plant derived proteins are of somewhat lower quality because they do not have the same balance of amino acids as meat, fish, cheese and eggs. They also tend to be short of vitamin B12, yet often contain more folic acid, vitamin B6, minerals and fiber than many meat protein diets.

For over 40 years, physicians have been victimized by "the great cholesterol con." It is still hard for some doctors to admit they have been deceived in personally avoiding whole milk, butter and eggs for so long, but the greatest hurt is that they counseled thousands of their patients to do the same.

Uffe Ravnskov, with his book, *Fat and Cholesterol are Good for You,*[4] joins Kilmer McCully in stating, "the only fats that are bad for you are those fats derived from polyunsaturated oils, like the corn oils of yesteryear and all similar products" (the ones that replaced our PUFAs). The saturated fats such as lard, butter, coconut oil, cream and animal fat that were consumed decades ago, are now popular once more, and deemed healthy.

References for:
Mitochondrial Mutations: Diet

1.Lee, R. *The Dobe Ju/'hoansi.* Thompson Learning Inc, 3rd, 2003

2.Allport S. *The Queen of Fats.* University of California Press, 2006

3.McCully, K. *The Heart Revolution.* Harper Collins, 2000

4.Ravnskov, U. *Fat and Cholesterol Are Good For You.* 2008

Mitochondrial Mutations: Diet
Chapter Summary and Key Points.

- Our Paleolithic days ended 10,000 years ago, but our bodies and metabolic functions are virtually the same as they were when our ancestors gave up the hunter-gatherer existence.

- The diet of our pre-agricultural ancestors consisted of meats, insects, eggs, vegetables, fruits, and nuts.

- The diet of the Greenland Inuit, who have a relative absence of heart disease, is essentially fish and seal meat.

- The blood samples of the Inuit were loaded with EPAs.

- Highly active, short-lived creatures have high levels of DHA. Large, slow and long-lived creatures have low DHA values.

- In our natural Paleolithic state, our dietary intake of omega-6 to omega-3 was about even at 1:1

- The ratio now is estimated to be 10, 20, or even 30:1.

- Food preservation and processing methods have diminished omega-3 because its unsaturated state makes it far more sensitive to oxidative change.

- Dr. McCully tells us that folic acid, B6 and B12 have vital contributions to the proper metabolism of homocysteine.

- Many vitamins, including the B complex, are often unable to function without adequate amounts of minerals such as zinc, magnesium, silicon and copper, and even other vitamins.

- Avoid canning. Freeze for storage. Do not overcook. These guidelines will give you optimum preservation of B6 and folic acid. B12 is much more stable and tolerant of heat.

The Statin Damage Gene?

What if today you awoke with the headlines screaming that 25% of the entire population of the United States, and a similar figure for Europe, carried a genetic combination that greatly increased their chances of serious adverse effects from the use of statin drugs? This is not just a bad dream.

With the advent of increasingly sophisticated and available genetic screening, much has been learned in these past few years directly bearing on statin toxicity. It appears that some of us are born with various genetic combinations that greatly increase our sensitivity to the various statin drugs.

A massive study out of Finland comparing Finns with the rest of the world has provided insight, chilling in its implications.[1]

This all has to do with a genetic combination known to geneticists as the *SLCO1B1* polymorphism, specifically the variant c.521CC genotype, affectionately known as "SNIPS" to workers in the field — special genetic combinations having very special effects.

This particular variant form has some rather remarkable effects on the pharmacokinetics (movement of drugs in the body) of different statins. Its greatest effect was on the plasma concentrations of simvastatin (Zocor). The 80 mg dose of Simvastatin has been banned through a black box warning on the drug by the FDA.

The c.521CC genotype has also increased the plasma concentrations of Atorvastatin (Lipitor), Pravastatin (Pravachol) and Rosuvastatin (Crestor), with significant but lesser effect on fluvastatin (Lescol), however, studies on the risk associated with these statins in individuals with the high risk genotype have not been as consistently reproducible as they have been with the 80 mg dose of Simvastatin.

Large differences in frequency of these genetic combinations exist between different populations. The highest frequencies of these variant genotypes were found in the U.S. (24% average, 18–32% range) with similar but slightly smaller figures for Europe (18% average, 14–23% range). The smallest frequency of this variant genotype was sub-Saharan Africa (1.9%average, 0.7–4.8% range).

This means that those in the United States are dealing with the presumed fact that 24% of the population are born with a super-sensitivity to statins, in that blood levels, following the usual dose prescribed by a doctor, are yielding values far higher than anyone expected them to be.

I have written before about the genetic complications secondary to statin use, but always with reference to mitochondrial DNA damage and mutations. Until I read this article, I had no idea that one-quarter of the U.S. population would be inadvertently super-dosed by statins because of a genetically programmed predisposition.

One would think drug companies would not let a moment go by before coming up with a test for statin sensitivity or, in accordance with the usual past practices, try to muddy up the research results and disprove the results and implications. Instead, the drug companies are trying to promote greater and greater statin use for primary as well as secondary prevention. Not a word about grossly adverse population genetics.

Although statins appear to be quite well tolerated by most people, twenty to thirty rhabdomyolysis deaths still occur annually from presently used statins, long after Baycol was removed from the market for just this reason. Peripheral neuropathy incidence is nearly as common as myopathy and most cases are permanent.

This toxicity of statins is a dose and concentration dependent phenomenon. This means that the risk of a toxic reaction increases as the plasma concentrations are increased. In my judgment, this observation demands an immediate investigation and even withholding of statin use until the 24 percent of the population at risk can be identified, but of course this will never happen.

Wide variability exists in the plasma concentrations of the cholesterol-lowering drugs in the statin class (HMG-CoA reductase inhibitors) as it relates to their efficacy and risk of adverse effects. The risk of muscle toxicity as an adverse effect of statin therapy is known to increase along with elevated plasma statin concentrations.

The gene, *SLCO1B1,* encodes (creates) a transport polypeptide (protein cluster) charged with the hepatic (liver) uptake of many endogenous and foreign compounds, such as statins. Because of the widely known diversity of the *SLCO1B1* gene from group to group, the goal of this investigator was to study the functional effect of this variability in the statin class of drugs.

Another mechanism exists whereby the potential of statin damage might be aggravated. Since statins exert their cholesterol-lowering effects by inhibiting the HMG-CoA reductase in the hepatocytes (liver cells), reduced transporter-mediated uptake in the liver due to these genetic abnormalities in *SLCO1B1* gene may also reduce the effectiveness of cholesterol lowering.

To the average physician, not getting the expected reduction in cholesterol means increased dosages must be necessary. So a 20mg dose must be increased to 40mg to get the desired reduction of cholesterol, or if already on 40 mg, it must be increased to 80 mg; further compounding the peripheral plasma concentration toxicity problem, and consequently the risk of systemic adverse effects such as myopathy and rhabdomyolysis.

The author of the study reminds us that in Finland, as in the United States, the six main statins in current use are simvastatin, lovastatin, pravastatin, fluvastatin, atorvastatin and rosuvastatin. More importantly, the author reviews for us their relative strengths. The roughly equipotent doses of these statins are: fluvastatin 80 mg, pravastatin 40 mg, lovastatin 20 mg, simvastatin 20 mg, atorvastatin 10 and rosuvastatin 5 mg.

Individuals, who cannot tolerate the higher doses when they could originally tolerate lower doses, may no longer be able to tolerate lower doses once they develop statin-induced myopathy.

Although much is made of the differences among statins, such as their increased water or lipid-solubility, they are all HMG-CoA reductase inhibitors; there are only so many ways this simple step can be blocked.

In the presence of such adverse events as cognitive and personality change, nerve impairment or muscle pain, rarely can substituting one statin for another provide benefit since they all do the same thing, using the same mechanisms. Any apparent benefit with a new statin is likely to reflect a somewhat lower dose, so a more productive option in the event of adverse response is dosage reduction of the currently used statin drug.

The importance of this wide range in strength among the various statins must be stressed. The strength range is very wide, with Crestor, the strongest statin, being 16 times more powerful than Lescol, the weakest, at the same dose. It is so easy for a busy doctor, frustrated by a lack of cholesterol response to Pravachol 40mg for example, to hurriedly switch a patient to Crestor 20mg, knowing it was stronger, but believing it was not that much stronger. The doctor has just quadrupled the original statin dose with hardly a thought. Crestor 20 mg is the same as Pravachol 160mg.

I know this sort of thing must happen again and again because of the excessively wide range of dosing now available. Now, into this pot of existing variability, comes this new information about how widely we differ because of genetic variability.

New genes with disease-causing genetic variants that act as risk factors for developing statin myopathy are being detected every year. Most of them are causative for underlying metabolic muscle diseases and are triggered by statins as well as by other environmental factors such as extreme exertion, exposure to heat, anesthesia, or viral infection. Therefore, in due course, even more than 25% of the U.S. and European populations may be found to carry genetic factors that place unknowing individuals at risk for statin-induced myopathy.[2]

References
The Statin Damage Gene?

1 Pasanen, M. PHARMACOGENETICS OF *SLCO1B1* : POPULATION GENETICS AND EFFECT ON STATINS. Thesis presentation to the medical faculty of the University of Helsinki, Finland. 19 December, 2008.

2. E.S. Stroes, P. Thompson, A. Corsini, **G.D. Vladutiu**, J. Armitage, F.J. Raal, K.K. Ray, M. Roden, E. Stein, L. Tokgözoğlu, B.G. Nordestgaard, E. Bruckert, G. de Backer, R.M. Krauss, U. Laufs, R.D. Santos, R. Hegele, G.K. Hovingh, L.A. Leiter, F. Mach, W. März, O. Wiklund, T.A. Jacobson, A.L. Catapano, H.N. Ginsberg, M.J. Chapman. Statin-Associated Muscle Symptoms: Impact on Statin Therapy. European Atherosclerosis Society Consensus Panel Statement on Assessment, Aetiology and Management; European Atherosclerosis Society Consensus Panel. Eur Heart J. 2015 May 1;36(17):1012-22.

The Statin Damage Gene?
Chapter Summary and Key Points.

- Many people have a genetic variant that greatly increases sensitivity to statins.

- The genetic combination is known as SLCO1B1 polymorphism, and more than 20% of the population in The U.S. and Europe may be affected.

- The toxicity of statins is dose and concentration dependent.

- Individuals who cannot tolerate a higher dose of a statin when they could originally tolerate a lower dose, may no longer be able to tolerate a lower dose once they develop statin-induced myopathy.

- Crestor, the strongest statin, is 16 times more powerful than Lescol, the weakest at the same dose.

- More than 25% of the U.S. and European populations may be found to carry genetic factors that place individuals at risk for statin-induced myopathy.

The Special Case of
Statin-Associated ALS

Neuroscientist V. Meske reported in the *European Journal of Neuroscience,* a relevant study about the ability of statin drugs to cause neuronal degeneration.[1] It seems that a consequence of the inhibitory effect of statin drugs on the mevalonate pathway, is the induction of abnormal tau protein phosphorylation.

Tau protein phosphorylation goes on to form neurofibrillary tangles, long known to be the prime suspect in causing the slowly progressive neuronal degeneration of Alzheimer's disease. Sometimes this process is accompanied by beta-amyloid deposition, but more commonly it is not. Research scientists are now finding that this mechanism appears to be true for amyotrophic lateral sclerosis (ALS) and many other forms of neurodegenerative diseases as well. They have even coined a new word for this, the tauopathies.

Statin associated tauopathies may well be additional gross evidence of collateral damage to existing cellular chemistry that researchers were unable to predict when they originally developed statins.

We have all been guinea pigs these past three decades. We were not told that these statin reductase inhibitors inevitably caused coenzyme Q10 loss, dolichol loss, and altered phosphorylation from mevalonate blockade. This implies that many statin users now are very likely to have accumulated adverse mitochondrial mutations.

At a meeting held in Salt Lake City, Utah from 21st to 24th September, 2010, Dr Benjamin R. Brooks, MD (director of the Carolinas Neuromuscular/ALS-MDA Center, in Charlotte, North Carolina) discussed in a video clip his study of 240 patients at an ALS clinic, of which thirty-one had been taking statins. Fourteen of these statin-using patients had a reaction to the statins consisting of pain and weakness, similar to that seen with myopathy in the twelve months preceding a diagnosis of ALS.

His study showed that use of statins with ALS patients may accelerate disease progression. Patients who are at risk from ALS, may have this condition occur more quickly in the presence of statins.

It would be interesting to see if other neurologists are reporting similar findings in their ALS patients because it would help underpin a much needed moratorium on statin prescribing in the presence of muscle pain and weakness.

The following link will take you to The People's Pharmacy website where hundreds of messages are available describing ALS or ALS-like reactions associated with the use of statin drugs.

https://www.peoplespharmacy.com/2009/07/31/statins-and-als/

You will note in some cases, these statin victims describe a PLS (primary lateral sclerosis) condition characterized by progressive muscle weakness, without clinically apparent atrophy. Many of these patients will go on to develop muscle atrophy, characteristic of upper motor neurone involvement in time, at which point their diagnosis changes to ALS.

We are seeing a spectrum of clinical conditions brought on by statin use, ranging from the pain and weakness of motor neuropathy and myopathy to primary lateral sclerosis (PLS) and atypical ALS. I strongly suspect the mechanism of action is mitochondrial DNA damage and mutation brought on by CoQ10 inhibition allowing excess free radical oxidation. Other factors must be considered, primary among which is the genetic predisposition from *SLCO1B1* polymorphism.

In my own research of some 10,000 victims of statin damage, I had noted a large number of ALS case reports which prompted me to communicate my findings to Joe Graedon of The People's Pharmacy, suggesting he may want to do a survey of his large readership.

In the year 2000, I had contacted Joe Graedon looking for any leads to my own statin-associated transient global amnesia reactions. At that time, the best that the medical community could do for me was to assure me that statins did not do that. He volunteered to post my query in his syndicated column. This resulted in a flood of responses from members of the public, and even doctors, not having the slightest awareness that statins could be involved in cognitive reactions such as mine.

Almost overnight we had 30 additional cases of transient global amnesia and hundreds of cases of confusion, disorientation, unusual forgetfulness and dementia-like reactions. Naturally, when neither patient nor doctor has the slightest awareness of a possible relationship between their new drug and cognitive symptoms, few if any MedWatch reports to the FDA are made.

Joe offered to start a special link, so people could post for others to see their own neuromuscular reactions to statin drugs. We both wondered what the truth would be with respect to ALS. Again, The People's Pharmacy column revealed the truth about statin associated neuromuscular degeneration cases, just as it had told the truth about the cognitive impact of statins that the medical community had missed so completely.

Since The People's Pharmacy first published their query in mid-2007, hundreds of email replies have poured in. I have a particular interest in this condition since my own muscular weakness problem was first diagnosed as ALS-like. My neurologist and I then considered PLS (primary lateral sclerosis) since I still had progressive muscle weakness, but with no evidence of atrophy or other upper motor neuron involvement. We were left with the conclusion that I was facing peripheral neuropathy.

References for:
The special case of statin-associated ALS

1   *Meske, V. and others. Blockade* of HMG-CoA reductase activity causes changes in Microtubule stabilizing protein tau via suppression of geranylgeranylpyrophosphate formation: implications for Alzheimer's disease. *Eur. J. Neurosci.*17, 93–102. 2003

The Special Case of Statin-Associated ALS
Chapter Summary and Key Points.

- Statin drugs have the ability to cause neuronal degeneration.

- Statins also cause the induction of abnormal tau protein phosphorylation.

- Patients, who are at risk from ALS, may have this condition occur more quickly in the presence of statins.

- We are seeing a spectrum of clinical conditions brought on by statin use, ranging from the pain and weakness of motor neuropathy and myopathy to primary lateral sclerosis (PLS) and atypical ALS.

- The People's Pharmacy column revealed the truth about statin associated neuromuscular degeneration cases.

Statins and Peripheral Neuropathy

I saw my neurologist in May, 2016, and he had concluded that regardless of my weight loss and obvious shrinkage of the muscle tissue of arms and legs, ALS, in his mind, just did not fit. The combination of tests he had done simply did not lead him to conclude that I had ALS, nor did he feel that further testing was necessary. The clincher was the muscle biopsy results, showing denervation atrophy of muscle fibers.

That says it very clearly, especially when combined with the results he got by sticking needles in the muscles and nerves of my arms and legs. Only one diagnosis could give the result I had shown — peripheral neuropathy. My nerves for pain sensation and my motor nerves were both involved, giving me pain and weakness, and somehow giving me the loss of balance which had been an issue from the very beginning.

Because of this imbalance, I had been referring to myself as an accident waiting to happen. It was such an obvious deficit; I was constantly on guard against falls. My neurologist said the loss of muscle was to be expected from the combination of age, and relative lack of exercise.

Neuropathy, short for peripheral neuropathy, simply means a malfunction of the peripheral nervous system that occurs without any inflammation of the nerves. There are many longstanding causes of neuropathy including diabetes, kidney problems and alcoholism.

Being placed on statin drugs is another more recent cause of peripheral neuropathy. Thousands of neuropathy cases have been reported to me over the years, and in 2012, FDA's MedWatch finally warned about peripheral neuropathy as a major adverse reaction to all types of statins.

The human nervous system consists of the central nervous system, which is just the brain and the spinal cord and the peripheral nervous system, which contains all the other nerves. The peripheral nervous system controls autonomic (automatic) functions of the body like breathing and heartbeat in addition to all sensory and motor functions, so symptoms may be widely diverse.

Muscle weakness is frequently a symptom of neuropathy and the muscle weakness may develop in a matter of days or may slowly progress over weeks or months. Individuals may simply not recognize the progressive muscle weakness and simply believe the symptoms to be the result of being tired, overdoing things or just getting older.

For those who take statins, keep muscle weakness in mind, for as the line at the end of the T.V. commercial, familiar to anyone in the U.S. warns, "it could be a sign of a rare but serious side effect."

Other symptoms of neuropathy include numbness, tingling and pricking sensations, burning pain (especially at night) and/or sensitivity to touch. Many people report loss of balance and incoordination. If left undiagnosed, neuropathy can lead to deterioration of the muscles and paralysis. Remember that we all need throat muscles to swallow, chest muscles to breathe and that the heart is a muscle. In extreme cases, severe neuropathy as a side effect to statin use can lead to death.

Some researchers estimate that 1 in 10 people who take statin drugs will experience a mild form of neuropathy where the symptoms may be a feeling of tiredness, difficulty in arising from a low chair or getting out of bed, shortness of breath, or difficulty walking. Cases of peripheral neuropathy, documented by muscle and nerve testing, have occurred from as little as a single dose of a statin.

Although some cases tend to improve in time after stopping the statin, the general impression from most doctors involved in trying to treat this condition is that it is resistant to all forms of treatment. In the past 12 years of monitoring some 2,000 patient reports, I have yet to find one who fully recovered.

Now we find that much of this statin associated nerve damage is sub-clinical, meaning that it is real, but the numbness and pain has yet to appear. This damage is below the threshold of clinical awareness, silently damaging unsuspecting patients.

The question of testing for statin drug damage must be considered by everyone experiencing adverse reactions from their statin. Common adverse effects reported by people taking statins are muscle weakness, pain, loss of ability to feel heat or cold, numbness and loss of balance. Sometimes these symptoms occur after only a few weeks of statin use. In other cases, years might pass before symptoms are noted.

In my case the symptoms came on several months after I had stopped taking statins for good. An important question is what testing should be done? How much testing is reasonable? In my own case my symptoms were pain in my lower back, weakness of thighs and loss of normal sense of balance. Gradually I noticed I had developed a stagger while out walking.

The first test my neurologist decided upon was creatine phosphokinase (CPK), and it was normal. The next test he felt justified in doing was electromyography, a test of velocity of nerve conduction in muscles after stimulation with a fine needle. Not pleasant, but informative. This was followed by a nerve conduction velocity test — stimulating a nerve with a fine needle, and measuring the speed of the nerve impulse as it travels down a nerve fiber.

The next test he recommended was a muscle biopsy, and he arranged to have this done by a local surgeon. A small piece of my gastrocnemius (calf muscle) was taken, which after staining, showed denervation and atrophy with both denervation and innervation changes. The final diagnosis after all these tests was peripheral neuropathy.

The usual drugs for neuropathy gave me intolerable side effects, with no improvement in my symptoms. In some 5% of cases like mine, the cause is an autoimmune process — important because treatment is available in these autoimmune cases. I did not have this test because it made no sense to me when one reviewed my history.

My first exposure to Lipitor 10 mg lasted only for three months before triggering my first 6-hour episode of transient global amnesia (TGA) causing me to quit the drug on my own. The following year on re-challenge (because statins don't do that, I was told) I was on 5 mg for only two months before it triggered my 12-hour episode of TGA. I quit Lipitor then for good. My muscle weakness, pain and imbalance came on gradually several months after I had stopped the drug. This is not the history one would expect from an autoimmune process.

A study in Denmark of neuropathy as a side effect to statin use, concluded that an individual who is a long-term user of statin drugs — two years or more — has a substantially greater risk of developing peripheral neuropathy than a person who does not take statin drugs.[1]

In two Adverse Drug Reactions Advisory Committee (ADRAC) cases of persistent peripheral neuropathy, motor and sensory conduction tests showed minimal recovery 4 and 12 months, respectively, after discontinuation of simvastatin, despite clinical improvement.[2]

A 2011 study (Otruba, P. and others), investigating the effects of simvastatin on peripheral nerve function, came to the startling conclusion that clinically insignificant peripheral neuropathy was occurring in all patients who had been on the drug longer than two years.[3]

Forty-two patients (23 males, 19 females, mean age 51.9 and 52.3 years) were studied. All were non-smokers and free of metabolic factors that might contribute to neuropathy. Initial examinations included laboratory and neurophysiological measures of the superficial peroneal and tibial nerves, focusing primarily on conduction velocity.

Treatment with simvastatin 20 mg daily was initiated. Patients were followed for 36 months with repeated neurophysiological examinations periodically during the study period. None of the patients reported such subjective symptoms as numbness or pain or loss of heat or cold sensation during the study period.

Despite lack of awareness of any sensory problems, repeat neurophysiological examination of lower-limb peripheral nerves at two years revealed gross abnormalities of conduction of both nerves. The authors reported that "long-term treatment with statins caused a clinically silent but still definite damage to peripheral nerves when the treatment lasts longer than 2 years."

References for:"
Statins and Peripheral Neuropathy

1. http://www.neurology.org/content/58/9/1333.abstract?sid=039a5bc7-0ece-4fd5-bae0-b6b8caefed8c

2. Australian Adverse Drug Reactions Bulletin.2005;24:6
https://www.tga.gov.au/sites/default/files/aadrb-0504.pdf

3. https://www.ncbi.nlm.nih.gov/pubmed/22167150

Statins and Peripheral Neuropathy
Chapter Summary and Key Points.

- My muscle biopsy results, showing denervation atrophy of muscle fibers, was clearly indicative of peripheral neuropathy.

- Neuropathy, short for peripheral neuropathy, simply means a malfunction of the peripheral nervous system that occurs without any inflammation of the nerves.

- There are many longstanding causes of neuropathy including diabetes, kidney problems and alcoholism.

- Being placed on statin drugs is another more recent cause of peripheral neuropathy.

- Muscle weakness is frequently a symptom of neuropathy.

- An individual who is a long-term user of statin drugs — two years or more — has a substantially greater risk of developing peripheral neuropathy than a person who does not take statin drugs.

Conclusion

Research literature is now replete with reports of mitochondrial mutations associated with the aging process, and many of the chronic diseases of aging, including such neurodegenerative diseases as ALS and Parkinson's disease. The underlying mechanism is oxidative damage — the consequence of energetic radicals striking adjacent mitochondrial DNA strands.

Now we find that statins affect mitochondrial DNA in the same manner by their inhibition of both CoQ10 and dolichols. The end result is premature aging along with its often associated weakness, incoordination and faulty memory, as well as increased numbers of neurodegenerative diseases.

The inevitable impairment of CoQ10 synthesis by statin drugs allows excess oxidative damage, and the similar inhibition of dolichols disrupts the DNA error correction process. The result is that not only do statins cause increased DNA damage, they also prevent its prompt repair.

The use of statins has resulted in the compromise of the dolichol and vital CoQ10 elements of the antioxidant system of countless people, resulting in seriously increased oxidative damage and DNA mutations.

The logical consequence of this is premature aging, and the progressive development of such chronic conditions of aging as muscle weakness, burning pain in the extremities, faulty coordination and failing memory — exactly the clinical picture we are seeing in so many statin users.

Statins drugs do have a small benefit for a few, but cholesterol reduction has nothing to do with this. The JUPITER study, that forever buried the cholesterol causation theory, proved to all thinking people that four decades of homage to the concept of cholesterol causation, was just a massive con.

Now we are seeing cholesterol sliding out and high-sensitivity C-reactive protein (CRP) sliding in as the only reasonable marker of cardiovascular risk level.

The fact that one quarter of the population of the United States and Europe is born with a genetic combination, greatly increasing statin toxicity, was stunning news to me.

Who among us, after four decades of brainwashing about the evils of cholesterol, would suspect its true role in brain function? We doctors were more like puppets to the pharmaceutical industry rather than partners in health care delivery.

Buried in the complex molecule of HMG-CoA reductase inhibition, is this special ability to reduce inflammation and modulate our immune system. We will find the key in time.

Duane Graveline MD MPH
Former US Air Force and US Army Flight Surgeon
Former NASA Astronaut
Retired Family Doctor

The Final Chapter

More than ten years ago, Dr. Duane Graveline began a series on spacedoc.com called *My Statin Story*.

Over the years, he chronicled his experiences and struggles with his own statin-related issues that began in 1999. You can find the whole of Dr. Graveline's account here:

https://www.spacedoc.com/articles/my-statin-story

Here is the final update to Dr. Graveline's statin story, which was narrated by his widow, Suzanne Graveline. It is a first-hand account of Doc's final weeks and days.

Dr. Duane Graveline - *My Statin Story.*

The Final Update, by Suzanne Graveline

August 2016.

For a month, I had begun to see very noticeable changes in Doc. Despite his difficulties in recent years, he always made a habit of going out for a daily walk. Not the four miles around the neighborhood with a backpack full of weights that he once did, but with the aid of his walker to help maintain balance, he was able to get some good regular exercise.

Recently he had cut back significantly on the distance he walked each day, and would now say that he was just going up to the corner and back. Neighbors noticed that he didn't have his usual spark and talkativeness. He would have his head down, not even noticing anyone, and his determined strides had become nothing more than a shuffle.

His muscle weakness was progressing rapidly. He had always enjoyed getting out of the house, and walking round the supermarket, and meeting and chatting with people, but now even that was becoming too much of an effort for him.

Doc was fully aware of these sudden changes, looking in the mirror and commenting on his physical appearance in particular.

The muscle wasting was accelerating. He had become skeletal in appearance. The bones in his arms, his shoulders and his ribs now stood out. His clothes had become too large for his frame, and his belts needed an extra hole added because his waist size had dropped so much.

When we went out together, he would always wear a jacket to help disguise the weight loss. Even using an electric razor became impossible because of the prominence of the bones in his face, so he went back to using a wet razor.

What was perplexing to us was that he retained a healthy appetite. He looked forward to his meals, enjoyed them and finished everything on his plate. But every day he weighed a little less.

In an effort to get some weight back on him, I started getting him some high calorie liquid shakes. He really enjoyed them — he liked the flavors and treated them like a dessert or a treat — and these were in addition to his regular meals, not as a replacement. Still he lost weight.

He had been having testosterone shots in an effort to get some muscle back, and these did get his testosterone levels up nicely, but there was no noticeable benefit to his arms and legs. Doc was pleased with the higher testosterone levels as he felt at least he was doing something positive.

He had been able to decrease his pain medicine by tapering down to lower doses and he stopped the pain medication patches entirely. With no fat on his body, it seemed pointless to him to be using them.

He was reading a lot, but also falling asleep a lot. The afternoon nap, that he had always taken, became earlier and earlier in the day until he was going for a sleep at 10:30 in the morning, and back again at 2:30 in the afternoon for another nap. The naps were longer and more frequent. He had also become very forgetful in the past few weeks.

Sunday September 4th, 2016

As always, Doc needed to be doing something, and he decided to take the garbage out.

I heard him come back into the house, followed by a thud, and I knew immediately that he was down. He had blacked out. I raced into his office and tried to get him up, but I couldn't lift him and he didn't have the muscle strength to do it on his own, or with my help.

He told me he was fine, said that nothing was broken, and he asked for a pillow. I said that we needed to call an ambulance, but he was very opposed to that idea because an ambulance meant hospital, and that was the last place he wanted to go.

I insisted that we had to call an ambulance, just so that they could get him back on his feet. He said that was fine, but only for someone to help him get up.

So I called emergency services, and both an ambulance and a fire truck arrived — Doc was not amused — but they got him up and did an EKG. One of the paramedics recognized Doc and knew of his medical training and experience.

Doc was insistent that he was fine and that everyone could leave, and no need to go to the hospital. The paramedic then showed Doc the printed readout of his EKG, and Doc said "Wow, I had better get to hospital now."

Doc was wheeled out to the ambulance, not laying down but sitting up. He looked pale and his skin was clammy. The hospital was the last place he wanted to go, but he knew he had no choice.

In the emergency room (ER), they first suspected a cardiac blockage. A specialist ran several tests. No blood clots. Arteries were clear with no blockages. No hardening of the arteries. His heart looked perfectly fine and healthy.

Nobody could see anything wrong. Doc still felt that the peripheral neuropathy he had previously been diagnosed with — by both his primary care doctor and his neurologist — was the cause. Doc was admitted to the intensive care unit (ICU).

Monday September 5th, 2016

While still in the ICU, he lost the ability to swallow food. He wanted the food, but just couldn't swallow it. His blood oxygen levels needed to be in the 90's, but his were stuck in the low 80's.

We were in ICU for hours while various tests were done. I asked Doc when he had last urinated, and he couldn't remember, so I said he should try now. He was only able to produce a very small amount, and it was dark brown in color.

A cardiologist asked Doc why he wasn't on a statin at his age. Well, you can imagine the look on Doc's face. He explained that he had peripheral neuropathy as a result of taking statins. Perhaps noticing a hint of doubt on the cardiologist's face, Doc said that he wasn't just saying this, and that it was documented with his neurologist.

The cardiologist said that there was a new drug now, an injectable cholesterol reducer. To this Doc asked if he reads much, and the doctor said not much because he didn't have the time. To this, Doc just smiled.

Doc told the cardiologist, "The disease has taken my skeletal muscle, so now it is looking for other muscle to go after." Doc simply pointed to his heart.

Thinking Doc might be more comfortable seated rather than lying down, they got him into a chair, but after just 20 seconds in the seated position, Doc was struggling to breathe. Still unable to find anything wrong, it was decided to keep Doc in the hospital another night for further monitoring.

Doc said to me, "Go on home, I will take a nap, and we will talk later. Either you can call me, or I will call you when I wake up."

I was only home thirty minutes from the hospital when the phone rang. I thought Doc must have rallied and was calling me to talk, but it was the hospital calling to say that he had died.

I feel that he knew exactly what was happening, and he didn't want me to have to witness it. Three days before the incident he told me, "I am losing my battle very fast now."

I dismissed it at the time thinking he was just hungry or wanting ice cream.

Doc absolutely dreaded two things, being a bed patient and any loss of his mental capabilities. Well he was never confined to bed, and mentally he was sharp to the very end, full of ideas and plans. Thankfully he was spared his two biggest fears in life.

Suzanne Graveline

Dr. Duane Graveline, Former US Air Force and US Army Flight Surgeon, NASA Astronaut and Family Doctor, died in hospital on September 5th, 2016 at the age of 85.

His ashes were interred at Arlington National Cemetery with full military honors on May 3rd, 2017.

His death certificate stated, as the causes of death:

a. CARDIORESPIRATORY ARREST

b. ACUTE MYOCARDIAL INFARCTION

c. CARDIAC DYSRHYTHMIA

d. PERIPHERAL NEUROPATHY

www.spacedoc.com

Made in the USA
Columbia, SC
11 June 2022